ISBN: 0-940258-16-1

Library of Congress Catalog Card
Number 85-80754

Printed in the United States of America
by Kripalu Publications
Box 793
Lenox, MA 01240

Kripalu Yoga

MEDITATION-IN-MOTION

Book II
Focusing Inward

YOGI AMRIT DESAI

"Kripalu Yoga is a Meditation-in-Motion, a pathless path, an effortless flow, a response to the primal wisdom of prana— with no techniques to perfect, no goals to be achieved, no routine to follow—a prayer without words, a divine dance— Kripalu Yoga is an experience of the moment."

Preface

This volume is the second of a series on Kripalu Yoga, a radically new approach to traditional yoga practice, created by Yogi Amrit Desai in 1970. In Book I, Yogi Desai described in detail for the first time the extraordinary personal experience that gave birth to Kripalu Yoga, after he had spent nearly 20 years mastering the art of traditional Ashtang yoga and was widely regarded as an authority on yoga. He described how suddenly one morning he entered into an ecstatic state of expanded consciousness, during which his body began to perform yoga postures automatically and spontaneously.

He recognized that this experience, which he called "Meditation-in-Motion," was the result of the awakening of prana (the intelligent life force within us), an integral part of Kundalini awakening. The prana thus freed in his body, together with his understanding of its workings, radically transformed both his whole understanding, perception, and practice of traditional hatha yoga, and his life.

In contrast to what is usually reported about such "peak experiences," he found he was able to reproduce these spontaneous postures again and again at will during his daily yoga practice. By studying the causative principles behind this experience he was able to develop from it a complete new yoga system to lead others towards similar experiences of Meditation-in-Motion. Whereas ordinarily, for successful meditation, stillness of the body is perceived to be essential, during the practice of Kripalu Yoga one experiences the paradox of simultaneous motion and meditation.

Kripalu Yoga is a holistic, integrated five-stage approach in which body and mind play a complementary rather than exclusive role. In Kripalu Yoga, hatha yoga postures are used not just as a physical discipline but also as a powerful method for actually entering into concentration and meditation.

In order to re-establish the original complementarity of hatha and raja yoga, Kripalu Yoga begins by restoring the cooperative working relationship between body and mind through specific techniques that particularly emphasize the importance of simultaneous pranayama (breath and life-force control) and concentration during postures. In this way hatha and raja yoga disciplines are practiced harmoniously and simultaneously. Body and mind enter into friendly union: the movements of the body are instrumental to the calming of the mind rather than conflicting, as in the traditional practice of meditation.

Thus in Kripalu Yoga body and mind, movement and meditation, and hatha and raja yoga are all simultaneous and complementary. From the very first stage, which is similar to the asana stage of Ashtang yoga, Kripalu Yoga begins to synthesize hatha and raja yoga into one holistic body-mind discipline instead of practicing them separately in a linear fashion, as is conventionally done.

The first volume gave an overview of Kripalu Yoga theory because understanding this theory is the key to successful practice of Kripalu Yoga, which is discussed in this second volume. Here in Book II, Yogi Desai describes the techniques for gradual awakening of prana through the medium of traditional hatha yoga postures and pranayama, and also a unique method for incorporating the more advanced practices of raja yoga into the practice of hatha yoga. This paves the way for Meditation-in-Motion.

Detailed instructions are given for daily practice of Stages 1 and 2 of Kripalu Yoga with the essential new characteristic of **focusing inward.** A subsequent volume in this series will provide practical instructions for Kripalu Yoga Stages 3, 4, and 5. Later volumes will each focus on one aspect of this multidimensional new form of yoga practice.

Because the knowledge contained in this series is not just intellectual theory and philosophy but the result of deep personal experience, it can be made an experiential part of everyone's life.

Contents

PART I

"Kripalu Yoga is a non-aggressive, non-intrusive, non-mental response to primal intelligence of prana working as the wisdom of the body. Even though it accepts all techniques and teachings of the great masters, its ultimate source for the guidance of postures is instinctive and intuitive knowing that transcends all limitations of both body and mind."

Classical Context of Kripalu Yoga

A Fulfillment of Patanjali's Ashtang Yoga

In the "Yoga Sutras" of Patanjali[1], there are two key statements which are central to the practice and philosophy of Kripalu Yoga Meditation-in-Motion:

1. *"Sthira sukham-asanam"*—*"Asana* (yoga posture) is that which produces steadiness and bliss" (II v. 46).
2. *"Yogas chitta vritti nirodah"*—"Yoga is the stilling of the thought-waves of the mind" (I v. 2).

It is usually assumed that stillness of mind is only attained through stillness of the body, as in seated meditation. Similarly, it is also assumed that yoga postures are to be performed separately from meditation, and what happens in the mind during practice of postures is often ignored.

And yet in 1970 I had an extraordinary and paradoxical experience[2] which revealed to me a whole new dimension in the practice of both postures and meditation, and which eventually led me to develop Kripalu Yoga[3]. During this experience my controlled, willful yoga postures suddenly changed into a flow of spontaneous, automatic movements carried out by an inner energy hitherto unknown to me. These movements were accompanied by a state of ecstatic meditation deeper than anything I had ever experienced before.

Meditation-in-Motion— A Synthesis of Hatha and Raja Yogas

I was able to re-create this experience day after day in my yoga practice, and as a result I realized that the popular assumptions that yoga postures and meditation can only be practiced separately and independently were incomplete. I had discovered a whole new depth and dimension to both hatha and raja yogas when they were practiced simultaneously. This experience revealed to me a radical new approach to the practice of yoga, in which both movement and meditation can happen simultaneously and be a complement to each other rather than a distraction from each other.

Kundalini Yoga—Prana Awakening

Those apparently simple statements of Patanjali I quoted at the beginning of this chapter clearly had a deeper meaning which suddenly had been revealed to me by my own direct experience.

I then re-examined the ancient, esoteric yogic texts and consulted with my guru, Swami Kripalvanandji, a Kundalini master, who confirmed that my original experience was an early manifestation of Kundalini *prana* awakening, as I had suspected. This all supported my intuitive knowing that I had rediscovered experientially the original inner essence and spirit of yoga through awakening the primal energy of prana, the life force[4]. Through prana awakening, that deep stillness of mind spoken of by Patanjali can be experienced not only in seated meditation but also during the actual performance of yoga postures. I also realized that, since Patanjali describes the whole purpose of yoga as "stilling the thought-waves of the mind," this must apply not just to the later "meditative" stages of raja yoga, but to every stage of yoga, including the postures of hatha yoga. Thus some degree of inner harmony, which is the very meaning of yoga, must be achieved at every stage of yoga, and not just be the goal or ultimate result after many years of practice. I feel that Kripalu Yoga is unique in incorporating these principles into its practices from the very beginning. Yoga postures become the vehicle for every stage of Kripalu Yoga, whereas in traditional Ashtang yoga they are abandoned when pranayama, concentration, and meditation are taken up as separate practices.

A Holistic Yoga for Body and Mind

This rediscovery of the original integral nature of hatha and raja yogas should not really be surprising, since science has also been rediscovering recently that our body and mind are not two separate entities, but are one holistic, interdependent body-mind. Every expression and experience of our lives is reflected in both our body and our mind. All our activities, experiences, and expressions are psychosomatic; body and mind act simultaneously supporting each other and influencing each other. When they are in conflict or are not supporting each other, our experiences and expressions are not total and are not ultimately satisfying.

Therefore our yoga practice cannot afford to be either exclusively mental or exclusively physical. And yet, in the traditional practice of yoga postures, very little attention has been paid to the role of concentration of mind during the practice of asanas; nor is the discomfort of the body taken very seriously during meditation. Quite often the benefits of hatha yoga are conceived to be limited to its relatively superficial physical fitness and relaxation effects. And yet the real potential of yoga is much more than these benefits of fitness and relaxation, which are available through the practice of any physical exercise.

Yoga Meant for
Total Spiritual Transformation

What makes yoga potentially unique is that it was specifically developed by great sages as a profound science for holistic and spiritual transformation on all levels. So while the benefits of yoga certainly include physical fitness and relaxation, they should never be limited to these.

Thus there are two aspects to the practice of yoga postures: the external form, the yoga posture that works through the body; and the internal form of yoga that works through the mind. Often in popular practice it is the external form, the technique, that is emphasized the most. The internal form—the attitude, intention, and mental aspect—is overlooked.

Until my remarkable experience, I had never imagined that there could be a technique in which the practice of hatha yoga postures could be used to greatly enhance the experience of the raja yoga disciplines of *pratyahara* (internalization of outgoing attention) and *dharana* (concentration) and vice versa, rather than restricting these to practice as separate disciplines, as is usually done. In Kripalu Yoga, the individual practice of hatha and raja yoga disciplines is certainly encouraged in the early stages, in order to master them. But only if each is performed with continual awareness of their ultimate inseparability will they lead the practitioner to the experience of Meditation-in-Motion, in which hatha and raja yogas coincide naturally and spontaneously.

Asana Itself Leads to
Meditation-in-Motion

This approach fulfills Patanjali's implication that the practice of asanas cannot be isolated from the true purpose of yoga. Thus asana is itself what "brings steadiness and stillness of mind," and "stilling of the thought-waves of the mind." So during practice of asanas, as much as during seated meditation, our purpose should be to still the "mind games": the internal chatter and endless inner arguments, the dialogs, conversations, comparisons, and complaints which so often form a part of our thinking, even during yoga practice.

So during the performance of Kripalu Yoga asanas, great emphasis is placed on becoming more conscious of the mental disturbances that are caused by the subtly comparative and competitive functions of mind that I call "ego-mind," because these disturbances are sustained by our lack of awareness of them. Yoga asanas are correctly practiced only if they fulfill the central purpose of yoga, which is the stilling of the mind.

From this expanded perception of the scope of yoga, and with a deep desire to share this ecstatic experience of posture flow with the many yoga teachers and advanced students I trained, I began to teach this new approach experimentally. Gradually over a period of years I developed it into what is now the complete five-stage technique of Kripalu Yoga. This method has three major purposes: (1) to transform traditional concepts of the separateness and linearity of hatha and raja yogas, and demonstrate that raja yoga is the essential, simultaneous, inner counterpart of hatha yoga; (2) to gradually lead the practitioner to a state of automatic, ecstatic postures and Meditation-in-Motion by incorporating meditative and concentration techniques into every stage of traditional hatha yoga practice; and (3) to provide a technique which will make the benefits of awakened prana, formerly only available through Kundalini yoga, available through the vehicle of traditional hatha yoga. This would then provide a third alternative or middle way to the previously mutually exclusive choices of Kundalini or traditional Ashtang yoga.[5]

Meditation-in-Motion Unfolds
All Stages of Ashtang Yoga Simultaneously

In my posture flow experiences I was spontaneously and naturally entering into all the stages of Ashtang yoga simultaneously: *asanas* (postures), *pranayama* (specific breathing patterns), *pratyahara* (internalization of the outgoing attention), *dharana* (concentration), *dhyana* (deep meditation), and ultimately *samadhi* (complete union with universal consciousness, in which there is no sense of the limitations of space, time, or a separate, conscious self). These stages are usually practiced in a linear, willful fashion; but in my case they unfolded one from the other in a natural, organic fashion, with each succeeding stage adding itself to the others, until all were experienced simultaneously in a peak yogic experience of self-transcendence. In this final stage of samadhi, movement sometimes continues, or the body may subside into complete stillness.

The "Inner Postures" of Kripalu Yoga

In Kripalu Yoga, mastering the postures is a necessary step, just as in every other form of hatha yoga. However, Kripalu Yoga emphasizes that the physical postures are to be considered as the external vehicle of the more significant "inner posture," which is the experience of complete inner stillness, harmony, peace, inner integration, balance, and union—which is yoga. This "inner" posture, which is Patanjali's "*sthira sukham-asanam*," remains constant even though the external postures are constantly changing. Thus the "stillness and steadiness" described by Patanjali as the main characteristic of asana is in fact an inner stillness of mind, rather than or in addition to the external stillness of the body as it is conventionally interpreted. This is why samadhi can be attained and maintained even during movement, and why in Kripalu Yoga the postures can play such a key role in stilling the mind. It is this internal stillness which brings with it the experience of joy and bliss, whether through external stillness or through movement.

Kripalu Yoga is a Spiritual Transcendental Discipline . . .

Thus in Kripalu Yoga the purpose of the asanas is primarily spiritual rather than merely physical. The external form of the posture is seen as secondary to its primary purpose as a vehicle for ecstatic, meditative experience. In this way Kripalu Yoga closely resembles the Zen approach, in which the particular art or activity being practiced (for example, archery or martial arts) is simply used as a vehicle for entering into deeper states of meditative consciousness to ultimately transcend the limitations of ego-mind.

So in Kripalu Yoga we use simultaneously both body and mind, both hatha and raja yogas, to transcend the normal limits of consciousness whose causes lie in both body and mind. So rather than the perfection of the external technique, which is important only as a vehicle, the focus in Kripalu Yoga is on internal perfection, which is mastery of the mind and awakening to higher states of consciousness. Yoga postures are thus seen as merely the external form through which the inner spirit or essence of yoga can manifest when the right inner attitude, purpose, and motivation are present.

. . . And a Continually Evolving Practice and Philosophy

I have developed this five-stage technique of Kripalu Yoga over a period of many years, continually refining each stage after observing the results of its application. During this process I have both closely observed the evolution of my repeated experiences of Meditation-in-Motion and also re-examined my original posture flow experience many times from many different angles. I frequently asked myself what the key elements were that had brought about my own experience. Each time I looked back, new insights emerged, which I have incorporated into Kripalu Yoga. This process is still continuing 15 years later (in 1985), and Kripalu Yoga is still evolving and becoming continually more refined.

In Book I of this series I gave (1) a detailed description of my own extraordinary experience; and (2) a comprehensive explanation of the role of what yogis call "prana," the life-force, both in my experience and in our daily life, in the workings of our body-mind-emotions, as well as its role in the creation and evolution of both the human microcosm and the cosmic macrocosm. In this second volume I have given a more expanded explanation of how prana manifests as what I call the "wisdom of the body," and how it is related to the practice of raja yoga during hatha yoga postures. I have also provided, in the second part of this book, a series of apparently traditional yoga practices, but I have also explained in detail how to perfom them in a way that will enable the reader to evolve toward an experience of Meditation-in-Motion similar to my own experience.

Some Comments About This Book

Because each stage of Kripalu Yoga is intimately related to an aspect of my own experience of the posture flow, I have felt that I wanted to include again in this volume a description of my original posture flow experience, because it illustrates in and of itself the essential principles of Kripalu Yoga philosophy and practice. I have also felt it necessary to repeat in distilled, synoptic form some of the earlier explanations of the role of prana in Kripalu Yoga, without which new readers who have not seen Book I will have difficulty in fully understanding what Meditation-in-Motion is all about. Those readers already familiar with this material will find many familiar concepts, but in the context of a different perspective, which hopefully will add a new dimension to your understanding. Naturally, if you have not read Book I and you wish to have an in-depth understanding of Kripalu Yoga, I highly recommend that you read it.

---

[1] Patanjali was the first to formulate the ancient yogic practices into an eight-step system called Ashtang yoga, comprising hatha yoga (postures and breathing exercises) and raja yoga (meditative exercises). The eight steps are: *yama* (moral self-restraints); *niyama* (moral observances); *asana* (postures); *pranayama* (regulation of breath and life energy); *pratyahara* (inward withdrawal of the senses); *dharana* (concentration); *dhyana* (contemplation); and *samadhi* (state of superconsciousness and bliss). See Taimni, **The Science of Yoga** (1975) p. 205. Full citations are given in the Bibliography at the end of this volume.

[2] See Chapter Two in this volume, and Desai, **Kripalu Yoga: Meditation-in-Motion** Book I (1985), pp. 23-27.

[3] Kripalu Yoga is named after Yogi Desai's guru, Yogacharya Swami Kripalvanandji. See brief Biography in the back of this volume.

[4] Thus my experience synthesized both the classical Ashtang yoga principles of Patanjali, and the ancient, esoteric, and difficult-to-practice science of Kundalini yoga. In Kripalu Yoga Meditation-in-Motion I have combined benefits of both in a series of practices that are both more alive and fulfilling than conventional hatha yoga, and less demanding and strenuous than Kundalini yoga.

[5] See Kripalvanandji, **Science of Meditation** (1977), and Desai, **Kripalu Yoga: Meditation-in-Motion** Book I (1985) for a full explanation and comparison of Kundalini yoga and Ashtang yoga.

"Kripalu Yoga is the expression of the inborn transcendental workings of prana, the instinctive wisdom of the body, the intuitive knowing of the higher self."

An Experience of Samadhi Reveals Deeper Potentials of Hatha Yoga

Pure Energy Takes Over My Postures

It is 1970. I am about to begin my daily practice in my house in Philadelphia, along with my wife Urmila and our friends Barbara and John. The sun is slanting in through the windows, its light dappled by the trees in my garden. In the background I can hear a tape of my guru chanting mantras, its gentle sounds awakening in my heart warm memories of his love and compassion. As usual, I am leading the group in a selection of traditional Ashtang yoga postures, carefully balancing each stretch with a complementary movement, as we move from Plough to Camel, from Shoulderstand to Wheel. As usual too, my attention is focused on the technical aspects of the asana, such as achieving the perfect alignment. My long experience allows me to enter into the postures with great ease, and I am gradually drawn deeper into the experience as my mind becomes ever more absorbed in the joy of moving and stretching my body.

All of a sudden I shift into a totally different level of consciousness than I have ever experienced before. I begin to feel waves of energy pulsing through my whole being. Without warning, urges are emerging that lead my body to begin moving on its own, entirely without my mental direction or choice. It is as if I am entering a whole new dimension of reality where every movement is effortless and spontaneous and my whole being is flooded with an ecstasy I have never known until this moment.

A New Ecstasy in the Midst of Motion

At first I am concerned about the others' reactions. I feel responsible for guiding their experience, and I don't want to leave them with any concern about what is happening to me. But I choose to trust this experience and their ability to assimilate it, feeling sure they sense the beauty of what is happening to me. As soon as I drop my concern for them, I am drawn deeper inside, and my body seems to become more relaxed and flexible than ever before, as it twists and turns through posture after posture, now slowly, now faster, now smoothly, now swiftly . . . I even begin to find myself in various positions I have never learned, even doing movements that seem not to be yoga postures in the traditional sense . . . I feel subtle tensions that I didn't even know existed in my body being released from the deepest levels . . . my usually active mind that normally wants to be in total control of my body has receded into the background, silently witnessing this amazing experience, noticing everything, yet not attempting to direct or censor the movements, nor making any critical, perfectionist judgment about my performance.

I feel as if I am watching myself from a distance, as if I am moving in a dream—and yet paradoxically I am more aware than ever before. It is simply that my habitual, mind-directed way of performing postures has been totally transcended, and I feel as if my body is being moved by a new and superior intelligence that knows even better than my conscious mind what movements I need to make, when, and for how long I need to hold them.

A Paradoxical Stillness at the Center

My ecstasy deepens. Now I feel as if I am at the center of the universe, moving in perfect harmony with everyone and everything . . . I have gone beyond all concepts of time and space, all relative reality; it is as if I am moving into the timeless moment of the Eternal Now itself. I am embracing infinity, where all dichotomies, doubts, inner conflicts, and limitations have dissolved into unity and freedom. Everything is paradoxical, yet perfect. I feel as if I am everything and yet at the same time I am nothing . . . I am full and yet am empty . . . I am active and yet I am totally passive . . . I feel as if my body, mind, heart, and spirit are fused into oneness. I understand intuitively for the first time words I have often read before, such as "effortless effort" and "choiceless choice" . . . I am no longer just doing postures; postures are happening to me and have become a doorway to a new dimension that reveals to me the mysteries of life. I am filled with ecstasy and bliss.

When I once again become aware of my body and surroundings, I am reluctant to end my blissful feelings by moving or even opening my eyes. When I eventually do so, it is with the greatest of difficulty, and only after two or three attempts. I have absolutely no sense of the passage of time, and I am amazed to find out that I have been unaware of my surroundings for over half an hour. With some concern, I look at my wife and friends; their faces, however, reveal a deep peace and blissfulness that seems to mirror my own. When we are all finally able to speak, I discover that they themselves were able to enter into deeply meditative states simply from sharing in the energy of my own process, and that they also had incredible experiences of seeing auric lights around me, and other paranormal phenomena associated with advanced meditative states.

I feel as if every experience I ever wanted to achieve through yoga and meditation just happened spontaneously without my having accomplished it myself—through some kind of divine grace or wisdom guiding me from deep within my body, far beyond the reach of my conscious mind.

The Awakening of Kundalini-Prana

Totally amazed at the whole experience, for a while I am at a loss to understand how or why this has come about. Then a brief but intense experience that I had had with Bapuji[1], my guru, in India when I was seventeen comes to mind. He had invited me into his meditation room to watch him during his Kundalini yoga meditation, breaking with the usual yogic tradition of maintaining complete secrecy of his sadhana. He had gone into a variety of postures and *mudras,* some familiar and others completely unknown to me, and afterwards told me that these were all performed automatically and spontaneously by the awakened prana. Naturally at the time I could not understand what that meant or how it was possible. Later Bapuji confirmed that my 1970 experience was one of the awakening of prana, which is an integral and initial stage of the awakening of Kundalini. The day after my first experience, and on succeeding days, to my great amazement and joy, I was able to repeat the experience.

I wanted to make this ecstatic experience

available to my advanced yoga students, so I began to explore the subject of awakened prana. I had never studied this in depth before, thinking it only applied to Kundalini yoga, which was not part of my practices (Bapuji had directed me to specific willful practices of Ashtang yoga). Intrigued and fascinated by the workings of awakened prana, I began to look for fuller explanations by rereading the yogic scriptures and esoteric literature on prana and Kundalini yoga, and also began to observe closely my own experiences. Through consistent study and practice, self-observation, and experiments, I was able to distill some of the esoteric teachings into a simple, practical system so that the whole dimension and scope of yoga that were missing in traditional Ashtang practice could now be made available to the sincere seeker.

Prana:
The Ultimate Inner Essence of All Yoga

Reflecting upon the significance of this experience, I realized that everything I thought I knew and believed about yoga had been changed. I saw that there was a whole new dimension to yoga that I had not perceived before. Until 1970 I had believed that in order to expand my experience in yoga and reach deeper meditative levels, I simply had to learn more about it intellectually and work harder at my practice. Now I saw that although this is true to some extent, this kind of externally acquired knowledge and practice is always incomplete if we do not have access to the inner intelligence of prana, that works both as the inborn wisdom of the body and as an innate intuitive knowing that comes from beyond all mentally acquired "knowledge". Clearly my body knew more about its own needs and how to meet them than any yoga book, authority on yoga, or learned technique could ever teach me.

I saw that what I described as the intuitive understanding of "effortless effort" and "choiceless choice" came from a source of primal

intelligence of prana beyond my conscious mind. It was the wisdom of my body that made the most perfect choices and then flowed with its own awareness effortlessly, without any intervention or disturbances from my mind (which did not need to know either how or why this was happening, any more than it needs to know exactly how to digest food or circulate blood).

My body's inner needs were the only criteria by which it selected the movements, and thus many movements were not even traditional yoga postures as such, but a variety of stretching or twisting movements, as direct responses releasing some inner tension. I saw I could draw upon this inner wisdom, which had so far remained dormant within me, as often as I allowed my mind to trust the wisdom of my body.

Continual Daily Revelations
of New Depths of Yoga

My experience of effortless, free-flowing postures continued day after day, as I was able to intuitively re-create again and again the specific internal and external conditions; and each time it was accompanied by a deep joy and fulfillment that I had never before experienced through yoga postures, even after 20 years of successful teaching and practice. After my experience I was more strongly drawn to daily practice, inspired by this daily experience of deep joy and satisfaction. My practice was no longer a dutiful discipline but a delightful and joyous experience. As I practiced regularly, I was able to enter into Meditation-in-Motion more and more easily. I would just close my eyes, take a few deep breaths,[2] and feel quickly drawn inward, as my body became deeply relaxed. Even when there were some external disturbances, I was able to disengage my attention from the outside world. As soon as my attention was focused inward, I felt my body getting urges to move in specific ways. Sometimes this inner urge to move was very pronounced and strong, at other times very gentle and subtle.

The Healing Wisdom of Prana

Prana even knew what posture to do to bring about healing in my body. For example, at one time I had severe back pain and was going to consult my chiropractor. I had tried to relieve the pain by postures that I knew to be good for the back. I was not only unsuccessful, but irritated the condition more. But as I relaxed totally and allowed this "wisdom of the body" to take over, it spontaneously did movements I hadn't thought of and released whatever was causing the pain almost instantly. Later I had several such healing experiences by trusting in the wisdom of my body to heal itself.

As I continued these meditative posture flows, each experience was one of total contentment and fulfillment. Every posture that the inner body urge guided me into was confirmed by my whole being. Each time I felt that nothing else could be more appropriate than what my body was deciding at that moment. Therefore there was no indecision or hesitation, which often creates tension in body or mind.

Ordinarily I would wonder which postion to choose next, and whether the selection was right for me. In the Flow, however, whatever urge arose in my body was validated by the total agreement between my body feelings, thoughts, and actions. They all said "Yes!" to each movement. There was no need for me to decide anything. The experience of joy itself, of total absorption and fulfillment—this was validation enough. There was an inner knowing that what was happening was truly in tune with my whole being. The deep meditation I experienced throughout my experience was further confirmation.

These experiences left no question in my mind: I was in the presence of some awe-inspiring higher intelligence than the mind. I felt that a divine, benevolent intelligence was guiding me for my highest possible good.

After I was well-established in this new-found way of entering into Meditation-in-Motion, I decided to share my experience with my advanced yoga class and the yoga teachers I was training. But since it was not the common experience, I found it difficult to explain to others in my class that there was an intelligence within their bodies that could perform miracles if they only could learn how to allow the free workings of this energy. So first I demonstrated my own posture flow. As with my wife and friends on the first day, they had some amazingly deep meditative experiences just from watching me.

Most people found difficulty in believing and expressing their experiences, as is often the case with meditative experiences, which are mostly right-brain, non-verbal and non-cognitive. They saw visions and lights, experienced spontaneous body movements, crying, feelings of deep joy and oneness—these were totally beyond the scope of reason and the logic of the left brain. The following are some of the reactions I received from them:

"My experience was one of observing pure energy flowing, changing and intensifying during the movements. Although there was no musical background, it looked like the flow followed a musical pattern. It seemed that each movement was naturally designed to occur in the sequence in which it happened. It was a radiant play of energy in motion."

"After watching you perform the posture flow I realize that I am finally seeing yoga in its pure form. I had done yoga before but my dedication would always come and go. I now see that when I was doing yoga before, it was more on the superficial level for its physical benefits. I feel I know the true, pure, and beautiful meaning of yoga experientially. I feel I understand more of its true origin and beginning as it was given to the first yogis. With this full and true understanding, come true love for the practices. I now feel a great love and total respect for yoga."

Amazed by the profound impact merely witnessing my posture flow consistently had on viewers, I continued to experiment with this new approach both on myself and on my students. I know that I myself had entered into this consciousness as a result of the awakening of prana. But I wanted to discover how to teach yoga so that anyone could begin to get some of these benefits and experiences from the very beginning, and at the same time gradually move towards the complete freeing of prana within themselves.

I found the most interesting task was to be able to translate these obscure, hidden teachings into terms and language that could be easily understood and incorporated into the practice of yoga in our own time. Thus began the development of a new way of applying the ancient teachings on prana to our health, our need for food and rest, to love, to healing, to our emotions and feelings—and incorporating them fully into hatha yoga in a way that can be both easily grasped and practiced by Western students. I continued to experiment with this new approach both on myself and on my students.

Kripalu Yoga Incorporates Raja Yoga into Hatha Yoga

So I devised Kripalu Yoga in five stages, a process by which the meditative aspects of raja yoga could be simultaneously developed within the physical practice of hatha yoga in order to accelerate the awakening of prana in a gradual organic way. With this process I hoped people could begin to have beautiful and meditative experiences of heightened prana activity almost from the start of their hatha yoga practice.

[1]An informal but respectful title for Swami Kripalvanandji used by his disciples. See brief biography at the end of this book.

[2]I used the Ujjayi breath desribed in the section on Pranayama.

"Kripalu Yoga is a paradoxical experience where opposites of effortless effort, choiceless choice, stillness and motion are experienced simultaneously."

The Results of My Kundalini Awakening

An Overview

My experience of the awakening prana was not just one of spiritual ecstasy and extraordinary psychic meditative states. This prana awakening permanently changed not only my perceptions and practice of yoga, but also my relationship to everything else in my life. I would like to share with you some of the changes so that you realize that Kripalu Yoga practices do not just touch the surface of life or part of life but in fact have the power to transform the whole of life.

Perceptual Changes

After my awakening, the world that my senses perceived seemed to have acquired new overtones, and I sensed words, sounds, sights, music, touch—the whole of reality—with greater clarity. I responded to the smallest details with a deep concentration that came effortlessly and naturally. Natural beauty was revealed to my senses with a new depth. Having been an artist for many years, I had always been very sensitive to beauty. But what I now experienced was not just an appreciation of beauty from an aesthetic, intellectual point of view that had been learned; I was feeling it more deeply than I ever had before.

My perceptions of other people had also deepened. It was as if I could sense and see, feel and experience, the subtler aspects of people's personalities. What had been invisible to me before became now very obvious. It was as if I could see through people's masks and facades. The slightest changes in tone of voice or choice of words revealed their inner feelings (whether guilt, fear and attachment, or love and compassion) with great clarity and accuracy.

Changes in Social and Family Relationships

Suddenly, too, my former patterns of relating to my social, familial, and cultural surroundings were different; they no longer held the same meaning as before. My value system underwent a profound change. My former interests and involvements were no longer attractive or alluring, and even when I did participate in them, I no longer felt any need to repeat them or form a habit of them. My attention was much more internalized than before, and so my involvement in external affairs declined along with my interest. This does not mean that I became aloof and withdrawn from the world around me. I simply felt more satisfied within myself, and thus had less need to look outside of myself for fulfillment or validation of my self-worth.

Whenever it was necessary for me to interact with external situations, I did so willingly as a simple, natural response to the esssential requirements of daily life. I looked at everything that I was doing and that was happening outside of me in relation to my internal growth. In this way, all my interactions with the external world and relationships became a way of seeing myself more and more clearly. I had never been a judgmental person, but I was somewhat idealistic. Now there was no longer any subtle, idealistic basis for judging myself or others on any score. I saw everything as simply cause and effect, with no blame anywhere for anyone. Any need to use traditional, conventional criteria for evaluating my personal growth had completely disappeared. I felt that I was "enough unto myself."

Internalization of Authority

In spite of all these internal changes, externally I continued to work within traditional social, cultural, financial, and religious structures. I remained responsible for the large yoga organization I had founded, maintaining all its necessary business aspects and conducting yoga classes, as well as meeting my family obligations, helping my friends as before, giving seminars and lectures, and so on.

The difference was that I no longer fulfilled these roles of father, husband, head of the organization, etc. to get even the most subtle level of confirmation or validation from society, friends, or relatives. Even before, I had been a self-sufficient, inner-motivated person. But now the last vestiges of need for social approval dropped away, and I felt completely free of all external constraints. I was not seeking any personal reward from these roles, but simply doing them because that was what I needed to

do at the time. Nothing I had to do was too big or too small for me to do. The distance between my usual daily life and spiritual life was quickly dissolving. I was willing to continue to relate to others in the way they needed from me, rather than to create a separation from them by insisting upon the perceptions brought about by my new state of consciousness. (Just as the external form of my yoga practice remained, but my whole internal attitude toward yoga was transformed, so also in my daily life my external activities remained essentially the same, yet my internal attitudes and concepts, personality and perceptions went through a profound change.) One external difference, however, was that I took part less and less in superficial conversations; these were replaced with more in-depth communications about core issues that more directly concerned my growth and that of others.

Most of all, I had the sense that I had found my own complete internal authority, which surpassed all conventional beliefs and dogmas. All the learned idealistic, moralistic, conventional, and traditional value judgments no longer had any grip on me. With that came a deep sense of fearlessness and freedom. Any former need to conform or to seek approval or acceptance was replaced by real internal needs and values that were directly and intuitively mine. When a need arose, my response followed effortlessly. My life flowed with the same effortless spontaneity as my postures during my formal practice of Kripalu Yoga.

Increased Nonattachment

Many other spiritual inclinations that had already been a part of my personality before this experience were now greatly accentuated. For example, I was even less attached than before to the results of what I was doing on the external level, and saw all interactions simply as tools for self-observation. Every activity was more an opportunity for self-discovery than it was work. My whole life was spiritualized. I truly experienced yoga as a way of life rather than a discipline with which to fight the nonspiritual parts of my life. As a result, my learning process, which happened through observation of my responses to external situations, became more acute and refined than ever before. I was able to use everyone and everything to reveal to myself all my strengths and weaknesses with great accuracy and objectivity.

Even though I was in love with and totally involved with everything I did, paradoxically I was able at the same time to witness it all with great objectivity and detachment. Usually when we are in love, either with someone or with what we are doing, we tend to lose the ability to witness it objectively. There is usually a tendency to develop a blinding attachment and even addiction in the name of love. The total involvement and love for life that I experienced after attaining this ability to remain consistently in the witness state reduced the possibility of my developing attachment and addiction. Love can be distorted by attachment until we have mastered the witness state. I was in love with life, yet I had no attachments to any of its pleasures. I was able to consistently work with them without getting caught in them.

Transcending Need to Renounce

Thus I felt no need to renounce the pleasures of life, because I saw that I had no compulsion for or dependence upon them, and was in no danger of forming a habit of that which was pleasurable. I could enjoy life's simple, natural pleasures and comforts, but I could also enjoy my life equally as well in their absence. To some extent these qualities were already in me, but they took a big leap at this time, and are continually evolving.

All these internal shifts were a result of the awakening of an energy and consciousness that ordinarily remains beyond the reach or grasp of the mind and particularly the aggressive ego-mind. It was an awakening of the core energy of Kundalini prana within me that simultaneously connected me to the core of existence—Prana—as well as to my own core. It was as if new internal connections were opened up that allowed my external and internal lives to come into harmony. I myself was simply the instrument in an uninterrupted process of internal transformation.

In this way, as a result of my prana awakening, my orientation to all life's interactions and activities underwent profound change. Thus the awakening of prana that revealed a whole new approach to the practice of yoga also led to the unfolding of a whole new expression of and approach to my life.

My Transformation Deeply Affects Yoga Students

The effects were very pronounced, visible, and obvious to anyone who had known me well before this experience. And this transformation had an equally strong impact on those I was close to, particularly my yoga students. My students showed and shared an unusual degree of openness and receptivity, reverence and respect for my teachings. Our interaction became more open. The degree of mutual trust and faith grew steadily. This was reflected in their lives. The whole atmosphere in the classes I taught became charged with a new feeling of reverence for the practice of yoga, of devotion and gratitude for the teachings. Somehow—without me telling them anything in words—my students attained new insight and depth in their own practices, which externally were the same as they had always been.

My own personal inner realization and transformation had become a catalyst for others to gain new insights into their own individual yoga practices. The changes in their own practice enabled them to understand my experience and its profound implication in my life. Their new experience of practice led to them to relate to me in a new way. There was a greater intimacy, a deeper level of communication on a direct energy level.

At first this experience, which opened up a whole new understanding of yoga, seemed totally unique to me, unexpected and unsought as it was. Then I began to learn of somewhat similar spontaneous ecstatic states of consciousness experienced by others in such diverse fields as dance, sports, athletics, art, music, etc.

Peak Experiences Compared

I realized that my own experience was somewhat similar to those referred to by Maslow and others as "peak experiences."[1] I realized, however, that my own experience and its follow-up differed dramatically from other such recorded peak experiences, in two major ways: First, I was able to repeat it as often as I wanted, and whenever I wanted; and second, I was able to develop it into a whole system so that others too could have such ecstatic experiences, rather than merely read about them or watch them, as is usually the case.[2]

Kundalini yoga is a precisely designed science, developed over thousands of years specifically to awaken energies and initiate such peak meditative experiences. These are not in themselves the goal of Kundalini yoga, but rather natural and predictable happenings during the unfoldment of higher levels of consciousness. As a result, the internal and external conditions that precipitate them have been systematically developed from the experiences of realized masters and therefore can be re-created.

Thus I was able to use my prana awakening in conjuction with traditional hatha yoga experience to develop a synthesis of the two. This synthesis would make the conventional, mechanical practice of hatha yoga come alive sooner by incorporating the wisdom of prana into it, and also develop prana awakening in a gentle, graduated way for Western yoga students who are not yet prepared to embark upon the more rigorous and advanced techniques of Kundalini yoga, which require great dedication and the supervision of a Kundalini master.

In this way, I would enable others to come to ecstatic experiences of deep meditation through movement, similar to my own, but in a shorter time than it had taken me, since the technique of Kripalu Yoga would be more focused towards that.

What, then, were those specific circumstances/conditions that came together to lead me into this extraordinary experience and enable me to re-create it effortlessly day after day? I referred to my own writings and some key phrases leapt out at me:

"I found limitless creativity was unfolding within me directly from my body. My attitude was more one of enjoyment, rather than of performing a task. *I was not trying to produce results or achieve the ideal that I held in my mind, or perfect the technique I had learned. I was completely at ease with myself . . .* "

I had not even realized that I had been trying too hard, because this attitude had been so subtle. What revealed to me that I was holding tensions due to "overachieving" during my previous practices was the contrast of the extraordinary new suppleness and flexibility of my body.

Reflecting on my continued daily experience, I had also written:

"Each time that I entered into the meditative posture flow, the more I abandoned my mind's usual need to control my body, guide its movements, and direct its course, the more my body became relaxed and moved spontaneously, uninhibited and free. I was trusting my body's wisdom to choose the movements and follow its own course of action. There was direct action: the feelings emerged and there was direct response from my body. There was only an awareness of actions, without interruption from the mind. *There was no interval between feeling and doing, urge and action—only an awareness. The inner became the outer; they became one.*"

Letting Go of Acquired "Skill"

As practice revealed to me new areas of wisdom of the body (for example, curing the pain in my back), my trust in my body's ability to make the right choices grew steadily. I saw that I used to do my postures exactly as I had read/seen in the book, and never questioned it. I held and increased the holding of the postures as books said one should. Although my body seemed to have no complaints, it probably had a lot to say about such regimented concepts, but I hardly paid any attention to it except when it was in actual pain. I gave it no chance to intervene in my mental plans for the practice. I was basically content with my practices, and had no idea what I was missing.

My new experience was thus a paradox: when I had tried hard to "achieve" a posture, I was not as limber and flexible as when I stopped forcing myself. I saw that the same principle lies behind the Zen arts, such as archery: for perhaps 20 years the archer studies formal technique in minute detail until eventually, without "trying," he can hit the bull's-eye even in the dark. Ballet dancers are also a good example—like Nijinsky, whose wife is reported to have said of him: "He just took a leap, held his breath and stayed up. He never could understand why we could not do it."[3]

Pure mastery of technique alone cannot account for these effortless and yet perfect performances, which seem to come from another dimension. And yet, without constant, dedicated practice, the artists could not have attained the mastery to transcend technique. It requires complete freedom from anxiety about technical points for prana to become free.

The same principle can be applied to hatha yoga, although traditionally it does not seem to have been. The dedicated willful practice of postures is intended to lead ultimately to the same freedom from all technique, but most traditional yoga stays within technique and is controlled performance. When we are still implementing learned techniques, it involves constant vigilance and therefore tension. There is a useful function to this learning only if it is a vehicle to transcend some subtle psychological limitations, and to ultimately let go of all reliance on external, learned technique and venture into the unknown freedom of prana.

This letting go of the mentally acquired technique enables your most creative spirit, the innate wisdom of your life energy, to be expressed. In Kripalu Yoga, postures are a tool for transcendence: you learn them only to ultimately let go of all you have learned willfully so that the inner wisdom of prana can take over. This is what happened to me during my experience, and the whole new approach of Kripalu Yoga is based upon this principle.

Role of Relaxation in Prana Awakening

Another important factor that I recognized as I observed my posture flows while developing Kripalu Yoga was the importance of relaxation in releasing the inner wisdom of prana in the body. I saw that there are many deeper degrees of relaxation within our reach than we ever realize.

When I practiced traditional yoga, even though my body would relax at a superficial muscular level induced by stretching, twisting, or bending as in many forms of exercise, the progressively deeper degrees of relaxation at the physical level, and even more at the subtle mental level, I see now, were not induced.

Even though I enjoyed the way I did postures before my flow experience, now when I followed the inner specific urges arising directly from my body and guiding it into various positions, I realized I was enjoying my practices even more because I was progressively entering into a deeper and deeper relaxation than I had ever sensed before. The deeper my relaxation the greater my prana release.

Prana: A Delicate and Sensitive Energy

Clearly, the prana flow is a most delicate and sensitive energy. I saw that if there was any force on my body exerted by my mind's demand for external performance, my body would obey, and prana's wisdom working through my body would remain suppressed and silent. In order to relax, I had to drop all expectations and be in a receiving rather than an achieving mood. If I was trying to force, master, or control it, the silent impulse of prana would remain dormant. Only when I was noninterfering—in the choiceless witness state—and receptive rather than wanting and forcing, did prana work freely. Tension in any form suppresses the subtle energy of prana, so in order to respond to the urges of prana, we have to become more sensitive. In order to be more sensitive, we have to be more and more relaxed.

I saw that what we normally call "relaxation" is a very superficial phenomenon, mainly concerned with relaxing the muscles of the body. In fact there are many progressively deeper levels of relaxation, both in the physical body, and also on the subtler levels of the mind. As we practice Kripalu Yoga, we gradually learn to penetrate these deeper and subtler levels of tension to relax more and more.

Gradually as each level allows the prana to flow more and more freely, the deeper states of meditation are attained. The spontaneous, prana-originated movements which occur then are rather like what happens when we are dropping off to sleep at night, and our body may jerk or twitch spontaneously as we relax and the control of the mind is withdrawn. The ultimate degree of relaxation is deep meditation, in which there is complete release of all tensions that arise from identification with body and mind. This develops a witness consciousness, or total identification with spirit, which is Prana. Even in deep sleep this does not normally occur—the mind usually retains some level of control over the body.

How Wisdom of Body Works

I saw that when I reached a certain depth of relaxation and sensitivity, the inner urges naturally released those specific movements of the body that were a response to my subtler, unrecognized needs for tension release. This is the function of awakened prana. Ordinarily the only spontaneous, automatic body movements we are familiar with are reflex tension-release actions such as yawning and stretching, a sudden urge we feel to crack our knuckles or neck, or to twist our back while we are in the midst of doing something else. It is our body's wisdom that takes care of those urges; such activities are not planned. We don't think, "Every two hours I will crack my knuckles or twist or yawn to work out accumulated tensions." It is just an urge that comes out of an unrecognized need sensed by the body; if the mind allows it, the body responds to its own need without our conscious control.

So relaxation is a progressively deeper and deeper phenomenon (in Kripalu Yoga) until the most subtle physical, mental, and emotional blocks and tensions are released through postures or other cleansing, healing *kriyas* (movements). Ultimately when the deepest level of yogic relaxation is achieved in dhyana and samadhi, the prana is released totally as in my Meditation-in-Motion experience.

When my body was deeply relaxed, I could feel and sense in the body the internally moving currents, or prana, and allow my body to move according to the inner promptings of prana. At such times my mind remained "actively passive." It simply attuned to prana without imposing its will or control over prana and simply cooperated with the inner subtle signals of prana. My mind became "passively active"; that is, it could also become active at any time and intervene if and when necessary to accommodate to the external conditions. But whenever my mind did exercise its will, its entry was most conscious and gentle so that it wouldn't disturb prana's flow.

During most yoga classes, when students are instructed to "relax," hardly anybody truly understands how to achieve that; the ability to relax deeply takes in-depth understanding, and explanation is necessary.

[1] Gallwey (1982); Gallwey and Kriegel (1981); Leonard (1981); McCluggage (1983); and Murphy and White (1978).

[2] Yogi Desai has taught the Kripalu Yoga method to thousands of yoga students and hundreds of yoga teachers since 1970 at Kripalu.

[3] Quoted in Murphy and White (1978), p. 104.

"Kripalu Yoga awakens direct response to the primal intelligence of prana working as the wisdom of the body. Its ultimate source for the guidance of postures is the instinctive, intuitive knowing that transcends all limitations of body and mind."

Kripalu Yoga and Prana

"Prana" and "prana"

For those readers who have not yet read the first volume in this series, I want to summarize the yogic concept of prana.[1] I will use *Prana* (with a capital *P*) to refer to the all-pervasive, intelligent energy the universe is made of, and *prana* (with a lower-case *p*) to refer to the part of the whole that is the life energy in each individual person.

It is the presence of Prana-Spirit that enables the body to absorb biological prana from the breath, food, water, etc. Just as breath is the life of the body, Prana-Spirit is the source of the life-giving breath.

The Universe Comes From Prana

Prana is the most basic and most subtle type of universal energy. The whole universe is created from the primal life force of Prana. Prana is the core energy from which all forms and forces of the universe have come into being. This Prana is the intelligent evolutionary life force that carries out all evolutionary cycles. Everything that exists in the entire existence is born of Prana, is sustained by Prana, and is transformed by Prana and again re-created by Prana in a universal evolutionary rhythm. The entire creation except man is governed by the natural, uniform evolutionary laws. Man is the only known being who has reached the peak of evolution and who can alter the evolutionary rhythm. Up to man, the evolutionary laws are self-governing. Man, the ultimate fruit of the creation, holds within him the seed spirit of the universe. This full-fledged expression of the Spirit-Prana allows him the freedom to realize the creator and be one with it.[2] This is man's inborn divine potential. This is why Christ says that man is made in the image and likeness of God.

Just as electricity manifests as light, heat, sound, and motion, etc., and yet is one energy expressing in multiple ways and operating through many forms, so also Prana, the life energy, operates and manifests in many forms through our life.

Prana is Our Life

The universal energy of Prana works through us as physical, biological, mental, emotional, and spiritual energies acting in our muscles, vital organs, nerves, glands, and brain. We draw and absorb prana through the medium of food, water, air, and sunlight. We store this energy in our glands and nerve centers. We expend our prana through our thoughts, feelings, and actions. We waste our energy through self-destructive attitudes and habits and through negative emotions such as fear, anger, jealousy, and greed. Prana works like a subtle electricity through the network of our subtle nerves *(nadis)*, providing the life impulse to the vital functions within our body. It nurtures our internal organs and intelligently carries out the most complicated vital functions such as digestion, circulation, respiration, elimination, and healing processes.

Such internal life-giving functions are carried out intelligently without our having to learn them. These functions we call involuntary are carried out by the innate intelligence of prana working through our body, aided by another form of prana's intelligence we call instinct.

Prana Functions at Many Levels

Prana's intelligence manifests at various evolutionary levels in human beings in the following hierarchical order:

1. In our body its energy automatically and autonomously carries out all life-giving involuntary biological functions, as we have said.

2. The same intelligence of prana also manifests as instinct that helps us to respond to all the sustenance needs for our survival.

3. Prana also manifests in its evolved form of intelligence in human beings as the mind, which helps us deal with all human needs in everyday life and explore our human potential.

4. Prana's intelligence acts as an evolutionary urge that constantly drives us towards realization of our inborn divinity.

5. Some of the transcendental qualities of prana's intelligence manifest through higher expressions of consciousness such as love, compassion, faith, intuition, witness, creativity, and psychic powers.

How Mind Evolved Control Over Prana

The first two levels of prana's intelligence, in which it manifests as involuntary bodily functions and instincts, are common to both animals and man. When this intelligence manifests at the next higher evolutionary level of mind, it has powers to override bodily urges, needs, and instincts. It represents a force that operates with greater scope and control than all that exists below the evolutionary level of mankind. This includes all that exists in the physical world.

plant life, and animal life. This is why the mind, the more evolved expression of prana, empowers man to understand and control all other manifestations of prana below it. This is why, through the understanding of the universal natural laws that govern the material world, man can manipulate the external world for his personal growth, comfort, survival, and pleasure, or explore higher human potentials through the use of his mind. We discover the existing laws of prana that intelligently govern the material world through various sciences such as physics, chemistry, biology, botany, zoology, geology, astronomy, etc, and exercise control over forces of nature and natural laws.

But this mind has its limitations. Just as the body or instincts can be overridden by the mind, so also the mind has its limits. Its functions are mostly limited to providing daily-life necessities. For effective daily living or for exploring human potentials, nothing can excel the mind. Yet no amount of mental powers and gifts of mind can reveal the transcendental power of spirit. Nevertheless, the mind is the only means we have to learn to go beyond the mind.

Ways to Transcend the Mind

The witness is higher than mind. So is love. If we want to draw upon the greater intelligence of prana, we have to learn techniques to transcend the mind. Various branches of yoga use various approaches and techniques such as raja yoga, bhakti yoga, karma yoga, Kundalini yoga, etc. to overcome the limitations of the mind, and ultimately to eventually transcend the mind.

The greatest of all limitations of mind, and one that keeps us from using prana's intelligence, is restlessness, disturbance of the mind. Fear, desires, attachments, insecurities, unnatural ways of living, violence, greed, and jealousy are some of the basic causes of mental disturbances. The basic purpose of Kripalu Yoga Meditation-in-Motion is to reduce and ultimately eliminate the restlessness of the mind, the cause of all inner conflicts, pain, and human suffering.

Prana—The Breath of Life

Prana is traditionally used to refer to the breath, because the life of the individual begins with the first breath in and ends with the last breath out, and is sustained by a series of uninterrupted breaths in between. Pranayama is a technique of using breath to master prana. Pranayama, or breathing techniques, are most powerful in controlling the restlessness of the mind. Breath and spirit are thus intimately related. In many cultures breath is conceived of as the spirit. The Hebrew word for "breath of life" can also be translated "spirit of life," as can the Latin *spiritus*. The English word *inspire* means "to breathe in, to infuse with spirit." The interchangeability of these two uses of the word *prana* represents the intimate relationship that exists between breath and prana.

The Evolutionary Potential of Prana

Yogis use postures, pranayamas, and other yogic disciplines to awaken and free the prana from the domination of the ego-mind. As I explained, this prana at its survival level carries out all vital, life-giving involuntary functions intelligently. Yogis have known the secrets of awakening the survival-level functioning of prana to the evolutionary level. The awakened prana automatically carries out physical, mental, and emotional purification at an accelerated evolutionary level with the same intelligence it carries out involuntary functions. Once the prana is awakened, it automatically carries out all internal purification and healing through postures, pranayamas, cleansing kriyas, and deep mental and emotional catharsis without having to learn them from anyone. The secret teachings on awakening prana in Kundalini yoga have been kept secret and revealed to only a few chosen disciples by the great masters.

The whole purpose of Kripalu Yoga is to enable us to use this intelligent life energy of prana for our own health, healing, personal growth, and spiritual evolution. This evolutionary energy has the potential to provide us with the same superhuman capacities, power, and strength that highly evolved saints and spiritual masters all over the world have relied on down through the ages.

Even though these secrets of prana have been consciously used by spiritual masters in other parts of the world, this tradition has not been developed deeply enough in the West to establish conscious scientific and practical techniques to tap into this unlimited wisdom that lies hidden within each of us. Kripalu Yoga makes this wisdom available in a systematic, scientific way so that it can be incorporated in daily yoga practice as well as in day-to-day life for well-being, peace of mind, health, and self-mastery.

All the disciplines of yoga, such as asanas, pranayamas, cleansing kriyas, locks, mudras, and concentration and meditation techniques are designed to enhance the absorption and storage of prana by improving our digestion, respiration, metabolism, and natural immune system, and by removing the restlessness of mind. This ability to consciously increase levels of prana actively working within ourselves enhances the sensitivity of our nerves, the workings of our vital functions, the clarity of our mind, and the balanced workings of our nervous and glandular system.

When your body is relaxed, your mind calm, and the survival instinct not actively working on meeting your survival-level needs, prana begins to work at the next level, which is evolutionary. When prana's signals become more pronounced urges, the body naturally responds to them. This is called awakening the wisdom of prana in the body. When there is no alarm for instinct to intervene, the higher wisdom becomes active.

Prana also opens a new dimension of intuitive perception that reveals secret knowledge not discernible through the five physical senses or conceivable through the reason or logic of the conditioned mind. This is why my own experience created so many inner and outer changes for me.

Kripalu Yoga Awakens Prana

Kripalu Yoga was born spontaneously from within as a result of awakened prana. By practicing it, anyone can learn to access this inner source of wisdom. So just as awakened prana was the source of the birth of yoga, yoga can become the source of prana awakening to ever higher and higher levels in body, mind, and emotions.

In describing my experience, I have said that my body moved spontaneously, effortlessly, and independently of my will—that up until this experience I had believed my mind to be the sole source of intelligence. Even though I knew from reading literature on Kundalini yoga and other scriptures that there was a "higher self" with "innate divine wisdom," that was only intellectual information. Then I discovered from my own personal experience the true nature of that greater intelligence that lies dormant within us. From this I developed Kripalu Yoga, which gives simple practical methods to awaken prana.

[1] For a more complete description of how prana manifests in the universe and in the human body, mind, and spirit, see **Kripalu Yoga: Meditation-in-Motion,** Book I (1985).
[2] See "God Is Energy" in **Working Miracles of Love** (1985).

"The purpose of Kripalu Yoga is to free the body from the tyranny of the ego-mind, which uses the body and yet often fails to nurture it, to support it, love it."

Ego-Mind and Prana-Mind

The Power of Mind

The mind is central to all aspects of our life. Almost all that is good for us and works for us happens through the mind, yet almost all that is harmful to us and goes against us also happens through the mind. Our mind is like water: it reflects the color of its container. It can be colored, taking on the hue of either the conditioned ego or the unconditioned prana.

The mind, which represents a special evolutionary gift to man, and which allows him freedom from the instincts that govern animals, is a relatively new toy with great freedom and power. Because of its advanced place in the evolutionary hierarchy, the mind has the power to be in tune with natural laws, to go against the natural laws, or to transcend these natural laws. When the mind goes against the natural laws, I call it the "ego-mind." When it works in harmony with the intelligent and natural laws of prana, working as wisdom of the body and intuitive knowing, I call it the "prana-mind." When the mind is used for exploring better health and higher evolutionary potentials, it acts as a friend and fulfills its true functions. But when the same mind is used to go against natural laws, it acts destructively.

Ego, Fear, and Survival

The self-destructive activities that suppress the evolutionary urge of prana and go against natural laws of health, love, peace, and harmony are the destructive acts of the ego-mind. Fear, anger, and self-rejection are not originally within us; they are the results of our going against our inner nature; the pure, inborn survival instinct; and our innate evolutionary urge. To the degree we seek validation from external sources, we are not in tune with the inborn wisdom of prana and cannot grow spiritually and evolve to higher levels of consciousness.

The body-mind's joint responsibility and highest priority is protecting itself from real threats against survival. Yet natural, instinctive urges that seek real safety and security for survival both in animals and humans get distorted when human ego-mind gains control of the same survival instinct, projecting false threats to survival and security.

Ego and fear are intimately related. The ego gains its strength and intensity from fear and survives through fear. When ego-mind projects unreal, false fears, the same body-mind under the influence of fear still reacts to these falsely perceived threats with highest priority.

Even though the mind has control over the body and instinct, when the mind is under the influence of ego it uses the body's energy for its own concerns. It is the fear in ego that makes ego so aggressive and that allows it to dominate the mind.

Conflict Between Body and Mind

Both the expression of the ego-mind and the expression of the prana-mind work through the same mind and create constant internal conflict. This conflict is essentially between body and mind.

Our body and instincts function in complete harmony under the natural laws of health. Yet the mind has the upper hand and control over body, and the mind usually gets influenced by the aggressive ego rather than the subtle, silent workings of the evolutionary voice of prana.

If the ego-mind gets into a habit or rut, the body mechanically acts under its influence. Thus restrictions in the ego-mind are reflected as restrictions in the workings of prana. All that influences the mind—personal beliefs and prejudices, likes and dislikes, changing moods and attitudes, fears and insecurities, cultural and social conditionings—also influences the body, because mind controls the body.

The basic purpose of yoga is to remove all restrictions and conditionings of the mind and establish body-mind harmony.

Kripalu Yoga teaches how to free the mind from the grips of the expression of the ego-mind to return through prana-mind to the natural laws and our inner nature.

The Voice of Our Evolutionary Urge

Through the same mind that we can tune into the natural laws of health and survival, we can also tune in to the higher evolutionary urges that help us develop high spiritual qualities. Thus the mind can be the vehicle to receive the spiritual gifts of intuition, creativity, psychic healing powers, faith, trust, and love. The purpose of Kripalu Yoga is to become more sensitive so that we uncover this hidden potential, this urge to expand, which is given to all human beings at birth, yet which can remain latent all our lives if we do not consciously awaken it.

Neither the instinctive urge for survival nor the evolutionary urge for realizing our divine potential are learned or adopted—they are inborn for the protection of our life and realizing our potential. But the instinctive urge has a higher priority over the evolutionary urge because without survival there can be no evolution. As we take care of the sustenance needs of the body, awakened prana gradually moves from this basic survival level to an evolutionary level, leading us towards our higher potential.

The inborn evolutionary urge of prana is the spiritual core of every human being. Compared with the strength of the instinct for survival and the power ego gains through self-induced fear under the pretense of survival, this urge is not assertive and dominating. It is subtle and delicate and yet it never dies no matter how long it is suppressed or ignored. It patiently awaits an opportunity for actualizing its inborn divinity.

The biological energy, prana, and the spiritual consciousness, Prana, are both transcendental forces available to us for the unfoldment of our inborn divine heritage. We have to gain access to both of these sources through the mind. This is why the mind plays the most important role in the practice of yoga. This is why Yogi Patanjali says "Yoga is stilling the thought-waves of the mind."

When the mind becomes steady and still—free from ego-motivated activities—it becomes clear. When the ordinary mind becomes transformed it begins to act on behalf of higher centers of consciousness. The still and steady mind can listen to the gentle voice that allows the inner intelligence of prana to flow freely. Then we begin to experience and express the transcendental dimension of Prana-Spirit in every aspect of our life.

"The practice of Kripalu Yoga takes place not just in your body but in your mind as well . . . its benefits are not limited by how stiff or flexible you are, by what your body can or cannot do, or by how well you have mastered the techniques or perfected the postures. Kripalu Yoga is a way to transcend all limitations and disturbances which infiltrate and influence every aspect and activity, experience and expression of life."

Identifying the Mental Habits That Prevent Concentration

The Wandering, Restless Mind

While we are physically engaged in any routine activity that doesn't require intense concentration, the mind tends to lose focus and roam around aimlessly from subject to subject. For example, we can attend more or less mechanically to the external details of driving a familiar route or cleaning the house while the mind drifts into daydreams and inner dialogues. The practice of yoga is no exception. Once we have mastered the basic postures and are comfortable with them, it is all too easy to lose our concentration and perform asanas mechanically, without much attention or awareness of the body, while the mind drifts away.

We miss an important dimension of any experience by not paying attention to what we are doing. But particularly in yoga we lose all of the subtler spiritual benefits—fulfillment, enjoyment, peace of mind—if we do not focus our attention fully on what we are doing with our bodies. Thus we not only fail to enter into the deep meditative experiences that are possible, we miss even some of the most basic health benefits of the postures, and may even harm our bodies from lack of attention. Here is a typical example that a yoga student provided one day:

"You were guiding us into the Plow, which is not very difficult for me, and so I went into it rather easily without having to think much about it. Then, as we held it, my mind wandered off and I started wondering what I would cook for dinner that night. By the time you told us to come down, I realized that my mind had been doing the shopping and planning the entire menu, and I hadn't even noticed whether the posture felt good or whether I was overdoing it...I realized too late that my back was really sore because I had held it too long without paying attention."

Watching your mind while doing the postures, and bringing it back gently when it wanders, is a key practice in Kripalu Yoga.

In addition to wandering thoughts, there may also be fear of failure, striving to prove oneself to others, seeking approval, projecting expectations on yourself, indecision, and self-doubt. All these thoughts and emotions create inner disturbance, reflected as physical tensions that prevent the prana from flowing freely. Observe your mind during yoga postures. I think you will begin to experience how any such thoughts, no matter how subtle, create an underlying tension in the body that prevents you from attaining to a more subtle meditative, inward experience.

Because I saw that the way I taught yoga before did not place enough emphasis on overcoming the usual tendency of the mind to wander aimlessly during the practice of asanas, I decided to emphasize awareness of inner mood and attitude, and how they affect the spirit as well as the practice of yoga.

Externalized Attention in Postures

By working with them more closely I came to understand that my students might have certain habitual thinking patterns that were creating subtle mental and physical tensions keeping them from focusing on their postures. It is ironic that there are such excellent books on how to make tennis or skiing more of an inner experience through using yoga techniques, and yet yoga itself is not being done with as much internal focus as it is intended to have!

During the actual practice of hatha yoga, little attention has been paid to the subtleties of inner attitude. Books and teachers usually teach in a general way that emphasizes the external aspect of yoga, and leave it at that. When we practice yoga, because there are no competitions, rankings, or awards as in sports and other physical activities, we may tend to fool ourselves into thinking that we are not practicing yoga in a competitive way, and yet the competitiveness is happening on a subtle internal level.

One of the other common attitudes that creates tension, striving, and forcing is excessive attention to perfecting external technique. Because of cultural upbringing with its competitive emphasis, new yoga students tend to compare their own "performance" with each other and wind up in a vicious circle of perfectionist self-criticism, self-rejection, more and more tension, inflexibility, and further self-criticism.

So I decided to get a few of my students to verbalize some of the inner dialogues and "mind games" that they experienced during class, as a way of helping them see the connection between thought patterns, physical and mental tension, and inflexibility.

If you have attempted yoga you will probably recognize some of these thoughts: "Should I be trying harder?"—"Am I performing as well as Jane?—I've been practicing for three whole months; when will I be good at the Lotus?"—"I wonder if my alignment is right."—"Is the teacher going to come over and correct/criticize me?"—"How much longer do I have to hold this? It hurts!"—"Do I look as good as the others?"—"My posture probably looks awful, not at all like the book." And so on.

If a teacher is constantly asking people to "correct" the postures, he or she may unconsciously encourage this kind of thinking, which creates inner tension and conflict. It is necessary to remind students that "perfecting" the external form is only a part of the posture—doing asanas is also a vehicle for inner awareness, a way to practice a different attitude toward everyday life. This invisible internal posture often remains unattended to and unnurtured, perhaps because the external form is easier to see and correct.

To facilitate focusing the mind and freeing prana through willful practices, the very first step is to become more aware of the tension-producing dialogues and habitual patterns that the mind normally pursues while the body is doing postures. So this chapter deals with awareness—with identifying the games of the mind during postures. Later chapters will focus on how to eliminate these mental distractions by practicing postures with focused awareness on each movement.

Typical Tension-Producing Mind Games

As I explored with my students the way the unfocused, undirected mind can act during performance of asanas, I came across various mind games having different causes and consequences.

The ego uses even yoga as a way to enter into self-rejection or competition if you start practice with high ideals that do not correspond with the reality of the condition of your own body. This sets the stage for self-rejection and fear, on which the ego thrives. It sets up an unattainable ideal of perfection.

If achieving perfect external postures is what captures your attention, many inner tensions and conflicts are created in the name of yoga, rather than reduced and removed. The whole purpose of yoga practice—the inner harmony and peace, the integration—is missed. This is the subtle internal part of yoga, which we tend to ignore. It is easily ignored, yet plays the most vital role in yoga. It is the core of practice. You don't have to perform a yoga posture perfectly in order to receive its full benefits. Such external achievement may show and prove to others your talent, may earn you awards and recognition, but no matter how spectacular and impressive, it has little internal value.

I noticed one day that a student of mine was close to tears, so I drew her aside. She told me she was in pain from attempting to do a posture that made her feel inadequate because she was too heavy and stiff to perform up to her level of expectation.

Judging and comparing ourselves to others, and then making critical judgments about ourselves has often been perceived as a way of improving our performance. When such criticism becomes exaggerated or generalized, it becomes discouraging, and if the discouragement and criticism continue, they become deep-seated internal blocks.

Depressed, frustrated, or angry, we are too discouraged to seek new, better, more creative solutions to overcoming our limitations. Some people believe that self-judgment is actually necessary. They wonder, "If I stopped criticizing myself, wouldn't I stop seeing my mistakes? How would I improve? Am I supposed to ignore my mistakes?" Letting go of self-blame and self-judgment is not ignoring or avoiding your mistakes. On the contrary, self-rejection and

self-criticism hinder rather than help our learning process. When we stop judgmental comments directed to our body, our body actually becomes more relaxed, more limber, and more responsive—which promotes a free working of prana.

Self-Improvement Without Self-Criticism

The best way to interpret your own limitations is the way that allows you to correct and improve rather than discourage and cripple yourself. So:

(1) Avoid labeling your performance at all, and particularly avoid calling it "bad" or "not good enough."

(2) Avoid comparing your body's ability with others', or competing with anyone by holding an unrealistic ideal in your mind.

(3) Do not exaggerate your mistakes. Do not generalize your self-judgments (e.g. from "I'm not doing this posture well" to "I'm terrible at yoga.").

(4) Describe to yourself what is happening with nonjudgmental awareness as it is happening, without bringing in any ideals or comparisons.

If you find some area in your practice where there is room for improvement without being self-critical, only then can you create appropriate conditions for self-improvement. And even if you catch yourself mentally evaluating your performance as "bad," you can still stay objective as long as you do not react emotionally. Whenever you have a negative, self-critical reaction to what you see in yourself, it creates physical, mental, and emotional tensions that undermine your ability to improve.

I am not saying do not stretch in order to improve your practice of a posture, nor be so gentle in your stretching that you hardly feel it in your body. That would be as inappropriate as stretching too much. So how do you know how far to stretch and when to stop? When does the pushing stop and responding begin? You know how far to stretch and push and when to stop and respond by relaxing during the stretch and listening to your body's signals.

The following conversation typically occurs in Kripalu Yoga training classes.

Yoga Teacher: "I want you to relax into the posture more."

Student: "But this is one of my worst postures. The Locust is really hard for me to do."

YT: "Perhaps you're trying too hard. Relax a little more."

S: "But if I relax I won't be able to do it at all, my legs will just fall down."

YT: "Of course don't let go totally, but just breathe into the posture, relax, and let go a little, then hold . . . see if that makes a difference."

S: "Well, yes . . . but it feels like my legs are hardly off the floor at all now. I had them up higher before . . ."

YT: "That may be true. You may have felt like you looked better in the posture, but the cost was too high—you were straining too much and that was counterproductive, creating more tension. Now that you've relaxed into it, see if you can lift your legs a little higher."

S: "That's funny . . . it's much easier to lift them up now than it was at first."

YT: "If you overstrain at first, you activate a mechanism in the muscles that locks them, makes them tense and rigid, and then there is no way that you can stretch to your full potential.

S: "It's amazing! I've been doing yoga for years, and I never would have believed that I could actually improve my postures by not trying so hard. I always thought that the only way to improve was to constantly push through my limits—like in athletics, for example, I would go that extra hundred feet, lift my legs up even higher . . . I almost can't believe that after learning this relaxed approach I'm actually doing better than I did before."

Overreliance on External Authority on Technique

Another way we allow our ego-mind to override our body is excessive reliance on external "authorities." I have noticed that quite often the printed word is equated in the mind with Truth. These ideas then have an almost hypnotic effect that overdevelops our trust in external techniques and philosophies, so that we tend to ignore or devalue the messages of our own body to which we are applying them.

When we learn yoga techniques from books or teachers, we must not forget that these techniques obviously cannot be designed to perfectly meet each individual's needs, with our different physical, mental, and emotional capacities. We must make our own adjustments to suit our own individual needs and capacities. Paying attention to the body and following its inner messages, in conjunction with following the learned technique, tailors the general form of yoga to your individual conditions and needs. Willful postures, practiced in this way, prepare for Meditation-in-Motion, which is totally inner-directed. Kripalu Yoga is an internal, personal form of yoga practiced in response to individual internal needs.

Thus in the practice of the earlier stages of Kripalu Yoga—the willful or learned practice—great attention is given to respecting, honoring, and trusting the body's needs, capacities, and limitations. The ego-mind must not lead us to impose force or violence upon the body, but instead to treat it with the gentle strength of relaxed attentiveness and awareness. At no time are we to ignore the wisdom of our own body, and fail to recognize its needs in favor of idealistic beliefs accumulated from external sources and imposed indiscriminately.

Trusting Your Inner Wisdom

There is another choice you can make to help you recognize your shortcomings, weaknesses, and so-called "mistakes" (which are simply false expectations) without blaming yourself. It works without your having to force or push for physical performance, thereby losing the very spirit of yoga. This other method is to shift to listening to the voice of your body's inner wisdom, prana. And in order to shift to inner wisdom, you have to learn to accept your limitations and strengths without fear or false pride, because judgment creates tension that prevents you from being sensitive to the body's intelligence.

In the practice of Kripalu Yoga the emphasis is on being aware of what is happening within your body, on attending to and responding to the sensations, feelings, and urges that arise in the body. The proper way to practice yoga is from love, not fear and judgment; enjoying, not forcing. This shift allows you to enjoy every stage of growth in yoga, instead of reserving joy for the end result while hating all that you have to do to get there. The joy comes from the *process* of growth rather than the end result. Yoga practice is supposed to promote self-acceptance, self-love, and inner harmony.

As you learn to trust this process, you become more relaxed and flexible, and the mind will let down its control and fears so that the body's wisdom may increasingly take over and facilitate the later stages of Kripalu Yoga.

As you develop a trusting, loving relationship with your body, it will reveal some of the inner wisdom of prana that will surprise you. You will find that your body knows more than you ever acknowledged or suspected.

"Kripalu Yoga is a technique that uses the classical hatha yoga postures as a vehicle to come in contact with the awesome power of the life force of prana that lies hidden within our body, mind, and spirit."

How Kripalu Yoga Differs from Ashtang Yoga

The Yoga of Will

Traditionally, there have been two formalized approaches to the practice of yoga: the path of willful disciplines, as practiced in the present-day approach to Ashtang yoga, and the path of surrender of mind to prana, known as Kundalini yoga. In the willful approach of Ashtang yoga, the mind is in control of the body. Any conditionings of the mind from authority, techniques, books, beliefs, culture, and society become limitations imposed on the body. These limitations restrict the wisdom of prana from attending to whatever is the priority for one's specific physical, mental, and emotional condition at a given time. Thus, even though the formal practice of willful disciplines may sometimes be a helpful guideline for the average person, it cannot be precisely tailored and prioritized to your individual needs of the moment. The purpose of Kripalu Yoga is to prevent the inhibiting conditionings and preconceptions of the mind from being imposed on the body, so that the inner, intelligent, healing energy of prana has the freedom to prioritize its own needs to suit your body.

In the West, the steps of Ashtang yoga (such as postures, pranayama, meditation, etc.) are usually practiced separately and sequentially for the specific benefits that are unique to each. For instance, postures or pranayama are usually practiced primarily for physical benefits, with no attention paid to the mind. As a result, even though the mind is in control of prana and decides what postures to do, when to do them, how long to hold them, etc., the mind soon becomes restless or bored and slips away into daydreams and fantasies. As another example, the meditative activities in traditional, willful Ashtang yoga are usually done in a sitting position, in which body movement is restricted or suppressed. In this case, it is the body's turn to become restless and rebel, as the knees ache, the back slumps, and the shoulders become tired. Thus, when the steps of Ashtang yoga are practiced willfully and separately, body and mind are constantly fighting each other. Inspiration diminishes, and to continue practicing one must often resort to a fixed, regimented discipline enforced by the clock. As a result, many people find it difficult to maintain the willful disciplines of traditional Ashtang yoga long enough to make in-depth changes in their lives.

The Yoga of Surrender

In the willful approach to Ashtang yoga, the mind exercises authority over both the body and prana. In the second formalized approach, known as Kundalini yoga, prana is free from any control of the mind whatever and conducts all purification activities (kriyas) on its own. In this path, the power of awakened prana overwhelms the mind, and the practitioner must be prepared to allow this intelligent energy to fully command his life. In this total surrender to prana, all ideas of right and wrong, of what is proper, idealistic and moralistic beliefs, etc., must be discarded—not only in terms of yoga, but also in social, religious, and all other areas as well. Because prana is fully awakened, the physical, emotional, and mental catharsis takes place at an intense, accelerated level. This catharsis is so intense that it requires great courage, determination, patience, stamina, and faith in guru and scriptures to continue. Those who choose this path must usually renounce all attachments to money, power, relationships, etc. Since the practitioner must be surrendered to whatever physical or emotional urges surface during this uncontrolled, cathartic process (such as bellowing, pranayamas, spontaneous postures, dancing, kriyas, chanting, laughing, crying, etc.), yoga practices must be done in seclusion. Thus, only a very few are capable of following the path of Kundalini yoga.

Kripalu Yoga: A Bridge Between Will and Surrender

Kripalu Yoga is a synthesis of these two approaches. It is a new method of awakening and heightening the evolutionary activity of prana that avoids many of the problems of willful practice; yet, it does not demand the extreme austerities of Kundalini yoga. In Kripalu Yoga, the mind is not in strict control of the body as in willful practices, nor is the mind completely surrendered to prana as in Kundalini yoga. Kripalu Yoga is a newly developed stage in-between, a fusion of the willful practice of Ashtang yoga and the surrender of Kundalini yoga, where mind and prana are harmoniously balanced. In a spirit of mutual cooperation, mind and prana contribute qualities and powers that are unique to each. Even though the life energy of prana has an intelligence that is far beyond the capacities of the logical mind, it cannot completely replace the mind when it comes to carrying out worldly responsibilities.

These two sources of energy—mind and prana—are like two wings of the soul. When we use both wings together, our spirit becomes free to soar beyond the limits of our logical, reasoning mind and to explore the hidden, evolutionary potentials that lie within each one of us. Thus, when we practice Kripalu Yoga, we rise to our fullest capacity while still remaining grounded in the world.

Steps of Ashtang Yoga

I have chosen to develop the new Kripalu Yoga practice through the medium of Patanjali's classical Ashtang yoga. Ashtang yoga consists of eight steps:

1. Yama[1]—ethical guidelines: abstensions
2. Niyama—ethical guidelines: observances
3. Asana—postures
4. Pranayama—breathing exercises, regulation of life force
5. Pratyahara—inward focusing of attention
6. Dharana—concentration
7. Dhyana—meditation
8. Samadhi—transcendental consciousness

The first two steps of this yoga are ethical guidelines that nurture and promote physical purity and mental peace, and thus greatly enhance the practice of yoga. Yama and niyama are to be incorporated in daily life within the context of both Ashtang and Kripalu Yoga; they are not considered part of the formal practice. Similarly, the eighth step of Ashtang yoga—samadhi—emerges naturally as the result of the appropriate practice of the previous steps. Thus samadhi is also not a part of the formal practice. This is why the formal practices of Kripalu Yoga corresponds with the remaining five steps of Ashtang yoga.

Kripalu Yoga—Same Steps, Implemented Differently

In the traditional practice you usually choose to master one of the steps at a time to the exclusion of the others. But in Kripalu Yoga, asana, pranayama, pratyahara, dharana, and dhyana are practiced simultaneously. Kripalu Yoga is first learned in five graduated steps, each of which places *emphasis* on one of the five disciplines being practiced while the rest of the steps remain subordinate. Stage 1 emphasizes asana; Stage 2 emphasizes pranayama; Stage 3 emphasizes pratyahara; Stage 4 emphasizes dha-rana; and Stage 5 emphasizes dhyana. However, all elements are present in each step.

For example, let us say you begin with Stage 1 of Kripalu Yoga, in which you learn the postures which you will continue to do throughout all five stages of Kripalu Yoga. Even as you practice the first stage of postures, you are guided to accompany the postures with deep continuous Ujjayi breathing, which is a pranayama. You are guided to draw your usually outgoing attention inward through breath, relaxation, and inward centering, which is pratyahara. Inward focusing on the internal experiences and urges in the body during your practices is dharana. All these various elements are present even in Stage 1. As you progress through the stages of Kripalu Yoga you become more and more proficient and focused within, until ultimately, all these steps are experienced fully and spontaneously as Meditation-in-Motion, the fifth and final stage of Kripalu Yoga.

Uniquely Flexible—Begin Anywhere

Because all these stages are organically and holistically connected, it is possible to start with any one, rather than be obliged to follow the traditional linear sequence of classical yoga. This makes Kripalu Yoga uniquely flexible and able to meet all needs of various personalities. For example, someone with a physical disability or a psychological disinclination to postures, which may have discouraged them from attempting yoga, can begin with pranayama; this may inspire them and later attract them to learn postures. And the same is true of any stage.

For some it may be natural to enter into the experience of Meditation-in-Motion without having practiced previous stages. Even if this happens to you, the practice of the earlier stages will help to deepen the final experience and help you to master it.

Enriching Ashtang Yoga

The practice of each Ashtang yoga step can be done separately as in the traditional approach, but incorporating the additional special techniques of Kripalu Yoga given below will greatly expand the depth and scope of each traditional Ashtang yoga step and also can benefit the practice of Kripalu Yoga.

Ashtang (Hatha & Raja) Yoga Steps	Special Technique of Kripalu Yoga
(1) Asana— Posture	Deep relaxation as focus of attention both before and during the practice of asana
(2) Pranayama— Breath and Life-Force Control	Continuous deep Ujjayi breathing during postures to keep the mind from restless wandering
(3) Pratyahara— Internalizing the Outgoing Attention	Extremely slow meditative movements that further slow down the mind and naturally induce internalization of outgoing attention
(4) Dharana— Concentration	Achieved during the holding of postures by focusing attention intently on the internal physical feelings, sensations and urges, and deepening and enlarging the scope of the healing and purifying power of prana through visualizations and affirmations
(5) Dhyana— Meditation	Remaining in choiceless awareness—witnessing all bodily feelings, urges, and responses to allow the free flow of prana through your body without censoring or restraining; remaining absorbed in the experience of inner harmony and unity

Dynamic Interplay of Hatha and Raja Yogas

The principles of hatha and raja yogas[2] are interwoven throughout the first four stages of Kripalu Yoga, which serve as preparation for Meditation-in-Motion. Raja yoga techniques of concentration are utilized from the very beginning to enhance the benefits of asana, unlike traditional hatha yoga. Hatha yoga practices of asana and pranayama are used throughout all stages of Kripalu Yoga, unlike traditional raja yoga, as a vehicle to bring the mind into the experience. From the very first stage of asana, techniques are provided to begin incorporating raja yoga techniques into the practice. Gradually the willful physical aspect is de-emphasized and the meditative stages of raja yoga are allowed to spontaneously emerge more and more. With each step the meditative aspect of Kripalu Yoga grows until at the final stage the flow of movement becomes the vehicle for entering into a deep meditative experience in which all first stages of Ashtang yoga occur spontaneously and simultaneously, as in my experience.

"The unparalleled beauty of Kripalu Yoga is that during its practice, asana, pranayama, pratyahara, dharana and dhyana are all happening simultaneously, not separately. Because Kripalu Yoga combines both hatha and raja yoga, it produces concentration of mind and steadiness for the body."
—Swami Kripalvanandji, *Science of Meditation*

This dynamic interplay between techniques for enhancing the working relationship between body and mind progresses to deeper levels at every stage of Kripalu Yoga. Because prana in the body is intensified by each of these practices singly, when they are combined a form of synergy occurs in which prana is greatly increased by the simultaneous practice of all these steps. This synergistic effect is what is missing in the isolated practice of hatha or raja yoga alone.

Asana—Stage 1

Even though the ultimate aim of Kripalu Yoga is to produce the experience of spontaneous postures, in the preparatory stages it is necessary to do willful, disciplined practice in order to learn the asanas thoroughly, just as it is in conventional hatha yoga practice. In any art or discipline, one has to first master the technique in order to ultimately transcend it, and in yoga it is no different. Postures are the foundation of Kripalu Yoga. Once the postures are mastered, other special disciplines of the later stages of Kripalu Yoga can easily be incorporated into your practice. The detailed description of the postures and instructions on how to perform them are given in Part II.

Pranayama—Stage 2

Pranayama plays a very important role in inducing deep relaxation and concentration of mind. In this stage you learn to practice Ujjayi breathing with the performance of your postures. A few other selected pranayamas are given, together with the instructions for their coordination with the hatha yoga postures.

A later volume in this series will include a detailed description of various pranayamas and their role in awakening prana.

Pratyahara—Stage 3

In preparing for the fifth stage of the Kripalu Yoga posture flow, Stage 3 is crucial to success. Here, the emphasis is on relaxing the body during the entire practice and moving the body in an exteremely slow, imperceptibly flowing manner. As soon as you incorporate these two principles in Stages 1 and 2, you are practicing Stages 1, 2 and 3 together. During postures, a passive mental attitude and deep relaxation of the body accompanied by extremely slow motion automatically creates pratyahara—withdrawal of disturbances entering the mind through the five senses.

"Once the seeker enters the stage of pratyahara, the rest of the components of yoga—asana, pranayama, dharana, dhyana and samadhi—are unfolded automatically in due course. That is why pratyahara is considered to be the point of entry into meditation, or yoga."
—Swami Kripalvanandji, *Science of Meditation*

The third stage is pivotal in Kripalu Yoga. Through the practice of pratyahara, you begin to control your senses, your powers of concentration improve, and your mind becomes sharp and focused. In addition, because your mind is focusing on pranic activity, it develops a heightened sensitivity to prana, which prepares you for Stage 4.

Dharana—Stage 4

As the mind becomes withdrawn from the outward disturbances coming through the five senses, it becomes extremely responsive to subtle urges in the body. As a result, the relaxation of the body and the calming of the mind release the blocks from the body, and the flow of prana becomes more intense and more readily perceptible. In this stage of Kripalu Yoga a special method of concentration is introduced that is designed to enhance the benefits of the posture. This is the technique of visualization and affirmation, which helps to accentuate the healing and purification processes integral to each posture.[3] By directing prana to the specific part of the body affected by the posture, by visualizing and affirming the physiological processes that are going on, you also develop your concentration, creative imagination, and will power. The more you develop concentration, the more easily you can bring your mind into greater inner harmony with the workings of prana.

Stage 4 integrates and enhances the benefits of all three previous stages. Thus, the first three stages become a vehicle for Stage 4, and the first four stages in turn become a vehicle for Stage 5,

Dhyana and Meditation-in-Motion. Stages 3 and 4 are designed to re-establish body-mind harmony. These two stages train the mind to tune even more deeply into the intuition, urges, and feelings that are the signals of prana working through the body. This body-mind attunement is the gateway to the flow of spontaneous postures of Stage 5.

Dhyana—Stage 5

After consistently practicing the first four stages of Kripalu Yoga, you will naturally awaken prana and enter into the fifth stage, in which postures are performed spontaneously and effortlessly as a Meditation-in-Motion. That yoga postures can occur spontaneously is an amazing concept for those who are only familiar with the traditional, willful approach to yoga postures. Nevertheless, if you properly practice the earlier stages of Kripalu Yoga in conjunction with proper diet and the right mental attitudes, you will arrive at this experience naturally.

The focus of attention of this stage is to allow the inner wisdom of prana to move your body—uninhibited, unobstructed, or unmanipulated in any way by the mind. At this stage, everything you have learned from books, traditions, techniques, and authorities about formal yoga postures and breathing exercises has to be dropped. You must learn to focus on only one authority: your own inner guidance. From this point on, there is only one book you will read for your practice of yoga—the book of your body.

Body-Mind Conflict Inhibits the Flow

To perform the flow, you must be relaxed and attentive to the urges, instincts, and feelings that arise in your body. In order to respond to the body's (prana's) urges, the mind must remain calm and passive. Ordinarily our mind orders our body what to do or what not to do. During most of our activities throughout the day, our mind is so used to exercising control over the body, that this becomes habitual. This makes us more and more insensitive to the urges and feelings that arise in the body. When we do respond to the urges of the body, we often perform movements mechanically and habitually; or because we are so busy with our mind-oriented activities, we even neglect these bodily urges and feelings altogether until they cause discomfort, tensions and pain. This constant tyranny of mind over the body causes tensions in the body which eventually become energy blocks. Because these blocks inhibit the flow of prana, we become even more insensitive to the wisdom of the body expressed as bodily urges, signals and sensations. This causes the body-mind split, where our psychic rhythms are in conflict with our bio-rhythms.

How to Perform Kripalu Yoga

The purpose of Kripalu Yoga is to remove energy blocks and to become progressively more sensitive and responsive to our bodily urges. In order to reverse the condition of tensions and energy blocks, your body must be relaxed, and your mind calmed. This is achieved by relaxing your body with a few deep breaths and by clearing the mind of any need to prove, achieve, force, or compare. Once you begin to move slowly into the Kripalu Yoga posture flow, keeping your body relaxed and your mind passive, the tensions will progressively diminish.

The energy blocks will slowly dissolve, and your sensitivity to the body's own instinctive inner urges will become more and more pronounced. The flow of energy will become freer as tensions reduce, and the body will begin to flow, move, turn, and twist—directed by the inner wisdom of the body.

When your body first begins to move with inner guidance at the early stages of learning to practice the posture flow, you will invariably question, "Am I making this happen, or is it happening on its own?" If you continue, eventually you will see more clearly the manner in which your body is moving. By and by you will become convinced that the unfamiliar postures are flowing with greater variety and combinations and that it is indeed your own inner intelligence that is behind the postures, rather than your mind.

Any disturbance at the level of the mind will cause tensions in the body and inhibit the flow, e.g. indecision, conflict, need to prove, seek acceptance or approval from others, fear, restlessness, etc. During practice of the flow, remain established in primal awareness (respond to the urges of prana). This can be done only if you let go of all preconceived ideas of yoga postures. Primal awareness is the state of choiceless awareness that responds to the inner wisdom of the body—prana.

We constantly abuse the body when we ignore the basic urges such as the body's need for rest, food, and elimination. We also do this when we ignore our body's signals and perform yoga postures or other exercises according to learned techniques, beliefs, and other's opinions. Many people who have forced their bodies to get into the lotus posture when their knees and hip joints were stiff or have continued to do the headstand when a stiff neck was protesting, have derived more disadvantages than benefits from yoga. The Kripalu Yoga way is to consult the book of your body first and not to impose or force your body to perform in ways that books, techniques, and authorities say you should.

Stage 5 is the Complete Expression of Kripalu Yoga

During Stage 5, you set aside all rules and restrictions that you have willfully practiced in the first four stages. Instead, you allow the posture to emerge spontaneously, guided by prana from within. These may be traditional yoga postures or even postures that you have never seen before in any yoga book. Do not suppress them if they occur, for prana is wiser than any book and knows exactly what your body needs at that particular moment. When you begin to do your postures in this way, a unique thing happens; you are now adding a new dimension to your yoga postures. They have become a form of Meditation-in-Motion, a prayer spoken with your whole being.

The Kripalu Yoga posture flow is an effortless, harmonious, rhythmic, balanced, and gentle flow of postures, and yet it produces inner stillness. The flow is guided from within in a meditative flow that gives a timeless quality to the movement. As you smoothly flow from one posture to another, guided by your inner energy, you begin to experience a deep feeling of balance and stillness. In spite of your body's movement, the inner stillness grows progressively until you become completely absorbed in the inner music of movements created by the harmony of body, mind, and prana.

As your mind begins to closely follow the inner guidance of prana, the mental and physical energies flow in attunement with prana and produce a meditative state of consciousness during the posture flow. Thus, the Kripalu Yoga posture flow is a very conscious experience.

---

[1] The yamas include nonviolence, truthfulness, nonstealing, nonpossesion, and continence. The niyamas include purification, contentment, self-study, surrender, and transformation.

[2] Hatha yoga includes asana and pranayama, which lead to pratyahara; raja yoga includes dharana and dhyana, which lead to samadhi.

[3] In a later volume on Kripalu Yoga in this series, separate and specific visualizations and affirmations are given for each posture.

PART II

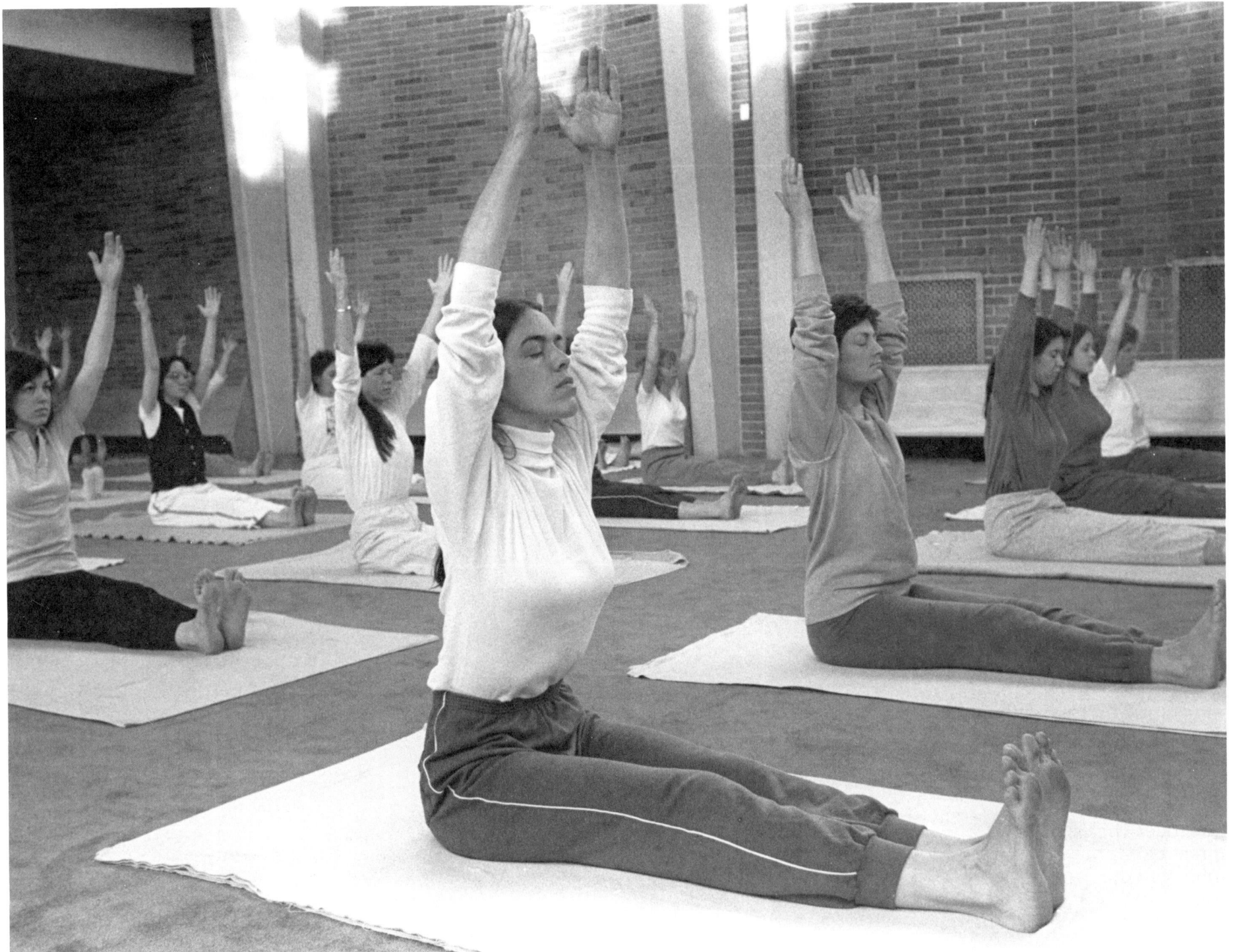

Kripalu Yoga: Your Daily Routine

Special Instructions for the Practice of Kripalu Yoga Postures

Remember that the purpose of Kripalu Yoga is deep inner transformation along with the more apparent external benefits of better health and a beautiful body. This internalized intention will give you focused, sustained strength as you go through the various stages of Kripalu Yoga, and will assure steady growth towards the ultimate experience of Meditation-in-Motion.

Various books and teachers of yoga differ in their description of the details of the postures, in their technique, and in emphasis. These differences in detail, approach, and technique are not as important as your inner attitude, trust in the wisdom of your body, and consistency in your practice. Do not let concern about such variations of technique and details of postures create indecision and doubt about your chosen practice. The purpose of Kripalu Yoga practice is primarily spiritual rather than physical, that is, inner transformation rather than outer achievement— awakening to higher consciousness

rather than perfection of technique, to the spirit of your practice rather than to the form, which is the only vehicle through which you awaken the spirit. Maintain the predominance of the spiritual purpose so that you do not get lost in the external details of the traditional forms of practice.

Even while practicing the willful stage of Kripalu Yoga, remember that patience, self-acceptance, and self-mastery are more important than the mastery of the technique or perfection of the posture. Make your practice of postures a vehicle for the practice of self-acceptance, rather than self-judgment; of self-love, rather than self-rejection. Use postures to overcome the restlessness of mind, not to create more of it through idealistic goals and anxiety about technique. In order to facilitate internalizing your attention during practice (in a group situation) keep your eyes closed as much as possible. This will help to avoid subtle competition or comparison with others.

As you develop in the practice of Kripalu Yoga, your practice will be guided and moderated more and more by the inner authority—your body—and less and less by the techniques given by external authorities. You confine the practice of Kripalu Yoga to a given technique in the preparatory stage only because it is specifically designed to facilitate the release of the spirit— prana—to replace the technique. In the final stage of Kripalu Yoga you let go of all acquired knowledge from external authorities so that the innate wisdom of the body—the intrinsic urges and intuitive inner guidance—may take over.

Kripalu Yoga focuses on practice rather than philosophy, on commitment rather than concept, on doing rather than thinking about doing. Consistent **practice** of this daily routine will carry you steadily towards the higher stages of Kripalu Yoga spiritual practices. I recommend that you set aside a regular daily time for your yoga practice and stay with it. Early in the morning before you begin your day's activities is the best time, but choose a time that is realistic for you in terms of your daily commitments. (If possible, practice your daily routine before breakfast; or else for best results allow four hours after a normal meal, or two hours after light refreshments.) I suggest that you commit the same amount of time each day, such as one-and-one-half hours, or one hour. However, if this is unrealistic for you, it is better to settle for less and to do it consistently than to continually fail to reach your ideal and become discouraged.

Preparation for your daily practice starts the night before with two very significant choices. First, eating a light supper rather than a heavy meal will help you wake up early feeling refreshed and ready to enjoy your yoga. Second, going to bed early (for example around 9:30) will make it much easier to get up early the following morning.

If you can, set aside a small room, or a corner of a room, just for yoga, and decorate it to create an appropriate meditative surrounding and mood for Kripalu Yoga. You may like to have a meditation table with photographs of great Masters and Saints—or if you have a Guru, with his picture—and candles and incense. You would naturally associate that place with your yoga, and it will build up the vibrations of your spiritual practices, so when you enter, you will easily be drawn into your practices. The place should be simple, clean, and quiet, with fresh air, and a mat suitable for practices.

Early in the morning, at a regular time, prepare yourself meditatively and lovingly to enter into the practice of yoga. Shower or wash so that you will be clean and comfortable. Dress lightly, and wear loose-fitting, comfortable clothing, that will not constrict your movements. When you enter your place for yoga, you may establish a meditative atmosphere by lighting candles and incense, and playing devotional music.

Begin your practice by centering yourself with a short meditation and by the chanting of OM. These serve to focus the mind and harmonize your energies. Then continue to draw your attention inward as you relax and calm your mind through deep Ujjayi breathing. Let your breath serve as a medium of concentration. Breathe from the abdomen and allow your mind to remain absorbed in the sound of the breath, bringing your full attention to the details of the complete Ujjayi breath for a few breaths. Then for the next few breaths, focus attention on the internal experience of breathing: the expansion and contraction of the lungs and diaphragm, the movement of the abdomen and chest, the flow of air in and out, and all the subtle accompanying sensations. This long, deep Ujjayi breathing should continue throughout the posture routine to help the mind be absorbed in the experience.

Throughout your practice, whenever you are disturbed by some external noise or by passing thoughts, bring your mind gently back again and again to your breath or to the experience of the posture that you are performing. Become aware once again of your movements and of the sensations produced in your body by the postures. Follow the Ujjayi breath (or other breath specifically indicated) as much as possible throughout the practices. When your body is following movements according to natural urges and you find some other natural breath patterns arising spontaneously, let them happen. If natural sounds of delight in stretching likewise emerge spontaneously, do not repress them. When you follow the natural breath and the sounds that arise, you are encouraging your body to express and regulate itself more freely.

Next move into 10-15 minutes of warm-ups to limber the major muscle groups in preparation for the postures; then proceed into the postures and the rest of the routine. Approximate timings for each part of the daily routines are indicated.

Cultivate pratyahara (withdrawal of outgoing energy) and dharana (concentration) during the practice of your postures by tuning into your body's internal experiences, urges, and sensations. This will internalize your outgoing, wandering, restless mind.

Anchoring your mind to your body helps not only pratyahara and dharana, but also opens up communication with your body.

During the practice be consciously attentive to the pleasurable sensations that arise from bending and twisting, stretching and relaxing, as tensions dissolve and release a flood of energy within your body. Let the delightful experience completely dissolve your mind. Let the sound of your Ujjayi breath, the expansion and contraction of your lungs as you inhale and exhale, absorb your mind. Watch yourself get off the merry-go-round of your mind as the body and breath draw you out of your thinking center into the feeling center, into the internal experience, the experience of the moment.

Let your movements be as if you were offering prayers to the divine. Let them be devotional, reverent, non-aggressive, gentle, and slow. This will further facilitate the slowing down of the mind and your receptivity to the flow of prana.

Pause after each posture and relax for a brief time. Observe your body being infused with newly released life force—feel the flow of the energy released by the stretch, squeeze, or twist of the body. Do not sacrifice the quality of your practice for speed. Graceful, harmonious, slow, conscious movements are the key to Kripalu Yoga.

Do not overdo a specific exercise just because you like it or can do it well. Rather, pay particular attention not to avoid those postures you find difficult. Remember, your journey begins from where you are now. See what your body can and cannot do, accept your limitations, and adjust the posture to your own capacity. As much as possible refrain from comparing yourself with others or worrying about what others will think of you. This will hold tension in your body, and reduce your flexibility. Remember that you are not pushing yourself to accomplish any specific goal.

At the conclusion of your routine, close with a meditation—extend it as long as you please. End your sadhana with a feeling of reverence, harmony, and gratitude.

ROUTINE #1
Preparatory Yoga Sequence 1

This routine is for those who have never done yoga before, or whose body is stiff from lack of this type of exercise. As soon as you feel your body is prepared, you can move on to the second sequence. The times given are merely suggestions.

Meditation (5 min.)

Meditation (15 min.)

ROUTINE #2
Preparatory Yoga Sequence 2

This routine is suitable for Beginners. Generally we recommend you practice this preparatory sequence for about three months, but the length of time may change from person to person. The purpose is to give you an opportunity to learn the classical postures, and to begin conditioning of your body.

Meditation (5 min.)

Meditation (15 min.)

ROUTINE #3
Kripalu Yoga Phase 1 Sadhana

This routine is for anyone. Generally we recommend that you practice this routine until you can comfortably hold these postures for one minute before you go on to Phase 2.[1]

Meditation (4 min.)

Chanting and Meditation

1. CHANTING OM or
   OTHER MANTRAS (5 min.)
2. MEDITATION (5 min.)
3. CHANTING OM or
   OTHER MANTRAS (5 min.)
4. MEDITATION (5 min.)

---

[1] It is much more beneficial to be trained in this routine than to learn it on your own. At Kripalu Center we offer a training program, which anyone can attend, which uses this sequence. There is also a training tape available from Kripalu Shop which leads you through the Phase 1 and Phase 2 routines.

ROUTINE #4
Kripalu Yoga Phase 2 Sadhana

This routine is for those who have practiced Routine #3 until they can hold the postures for one minute. The times indicated are merely suggestions.

Meditation (4 min.)

Bandhas and Kriyas (10 min.)

Meditation

1. MEDITATION (10 min.)

2. CHANTING OM or
   OTHER MANTRAS (5 min.)

3. MEDITATION (5 min.)

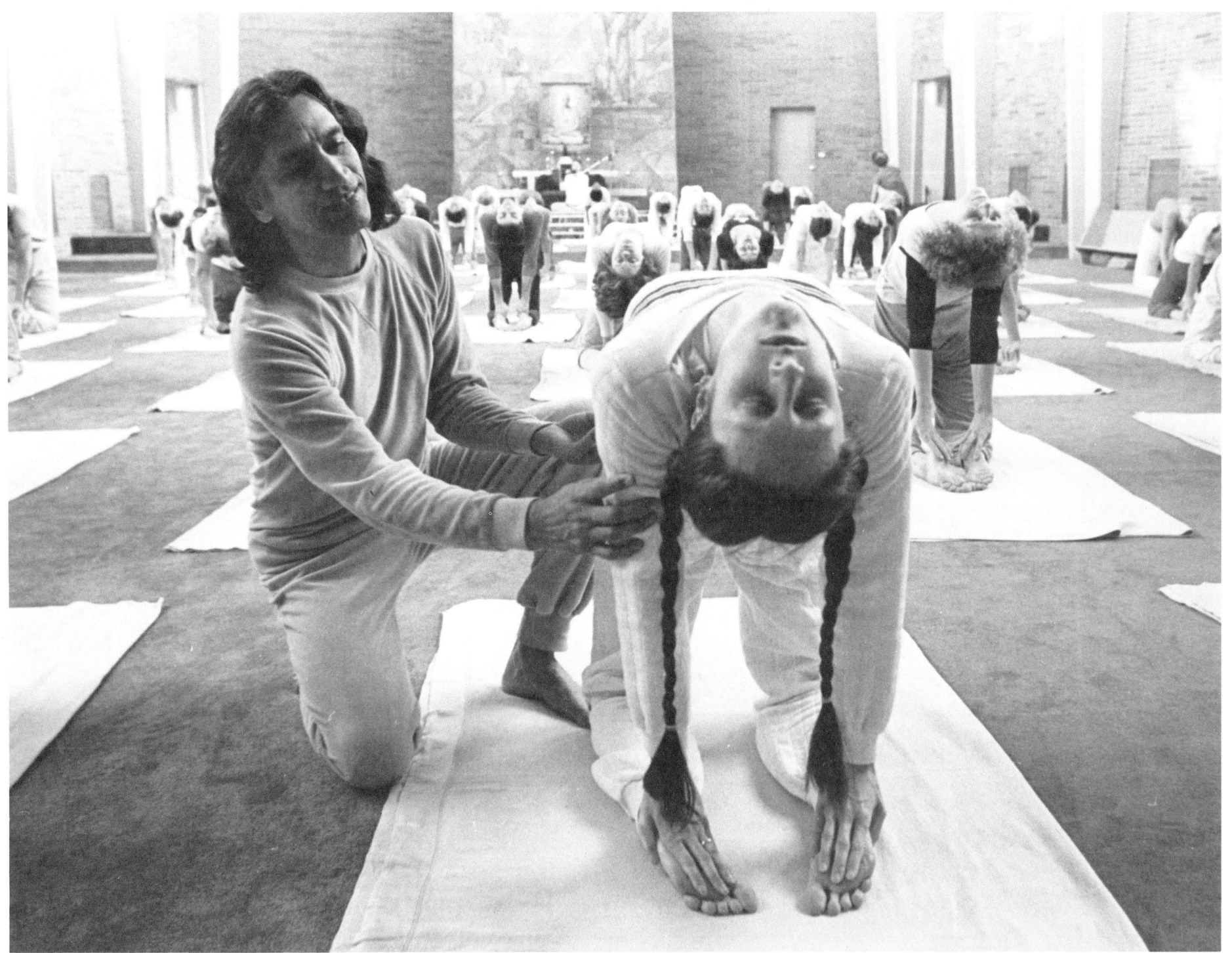

Kripalu Yoga: Postures

General Instructions for the Practice of Traditional Postures

The following instructions are to teach you the traditional postures. In Kripalu Yoga you learn to do the traditional yoga postures well since they are the vehicle for Meditation-in-Motion. Once you have thoroughly learned the posture, you gradually incorporate new elements of Kripalu Yoga to deepen your practice.

Read the description of the posture before you begin. Each posture is described step-by-step: both how to get into the final pose and how to release the pose. Special care is taken to describe proper body alignment when appropriate. Examine the photographs and notice the details of alignment. The focus on alignment will help you to keep your mind on the body, to avoid injury and undue strain, as well as to receive the most benefit.

As you first learn the postures, practice them individually before you put them together in a sequence, and focus your attention on the techniques necessary to assume the posture as described. Add no more than one new posture a day. Do each posture gently, with full consideration for your body. In the beginning, hold each posture for 10 seconds, gradually building endurance and extending the holding time to at least one minute.

While you hold the posture, pay attention to and breathe into the natural stretch-pain in the active part of your body so that you do not overstrain. Allow just enough tension-pain so that you can relax it consciously as you hold the position. Use micro-movements to remove hidden tensions. As you consciously relax you will release deeper tensions. As you relax specific areas, the blood flows more freely and carries away toxins, and at the same time new healing energy brings new life to the deprived, neglected, and sluggish areas of your body. Enjoy doing each stretch, and listen to your body as you do so. The enjoyable sensation and even trembling of a good stretch can be held, using long, deep breathing to allow the muscles being stretched to fully lengthen. Avoid sudden, jerky, or bouncy movements (which actually shorten and tighten muscles instead), and avoid any rapid movement that causes sudden, sharp pains. You will be amazed to see how your flexibility increases through gentle stretching done consistently over a period of time.

Coordinating Breath With Movement

Once you feel proficient in each movement, coordinate it with the suggested sequence of breaths. (The suggested breathing patterns to accompany each step are indicated to the right, in a separate column. The details of the breathing technique are given in the section following the postures.) Inhalations and exhalations have been specifically indicated to allow the posture to flow more easily and to enable you to move more naturally in and out of the pose.

The general breath coordination rules for postures are: exhale when you bend forward, inhale when you bend backward. Exhale every time you contract, twist, or squeeze your lungs and diaphragm in a movement, and inhale every time you open and expand your lungs and diaphragm. While you hold a posture, or when the breath is not indicated, breathe normally. Always breathe through both nostrils during all asanas unless specifically directed otherwise. Do not allow your breath to become forced or strained at any time during postures.

The mastery of the Ujjayi breathing technique is essential. Study and master this technique separately, then integrate it with your postures. Practice coordination of breath and body movements until you are able to coordinate your breath and movement without strain.

A Note for Women

Menstruation is a natural cleansing process for a woman's body. To allow this cleansing to happen naturally and to allow the body's wastes to be removed, it is important to avoid doing any inverted poses or strenuous pranayama techniques during the menstrual period. During menstruation continue to do all other postures in the sequence, especially those stated as beneficial for cramps, backache, and other menstrual disorders.

Exercise during pregnancy is important and beneficial to well-being. After the first trimester (the third month), postures that require lying on your stomach, such as the Cobra or Locust, should be avoided; also any posture requiring added pressure to the abdomen, such as the Peacock or Abdominal Massage; and any forward-bending posture, such as the Yoga Mudra, and the Forward Bend. Backward-bending postures should be done only by those women who have consulted their physicians and who are advanced in the practice of yoga. The only pranayamas to practice during pregnancy are Ujjayi and Anulom Viloma. Others should be avoided.

Consult your doctor before taking up yoga practices if you have any unusual health or pregnancy conditions.

WARM-UPS

These exercises are to warm the body and limber the muscles for the more strenuous stretching and holding of the yoga postures. Keep moving to stimulate circulation and respiration. Ten to fifteen minutes may be used for warm-ups before each yoga session.

For dynamic exercises such as the Trapeze, the Standing Squats, and the Airplane, the breathing pattern should be deep inhalations and forceful exhalations through the mouth. This vigorous breathing further helps the muscles to warm up in preparation for the postures.

Neck Stretches

1. Stand up. Drop chin forward to chest.

2. Slowly lift head up and back, then slowly forward. Repeat 3-5 times.

3. Tip the head to the right. Slowly lift the head up and tip to the left. Raise the head back to center. Repeat 3-5 times.

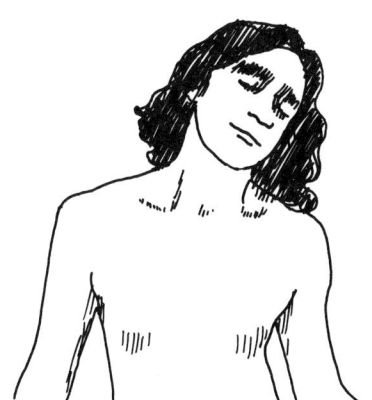

Standing Swinging Twists

1. Stand with feet several inches wider than hip-width apart.

2. Swing arms from side to side, originating the movement from your hips.

3. Turn head to look in direction of your swinging arms.

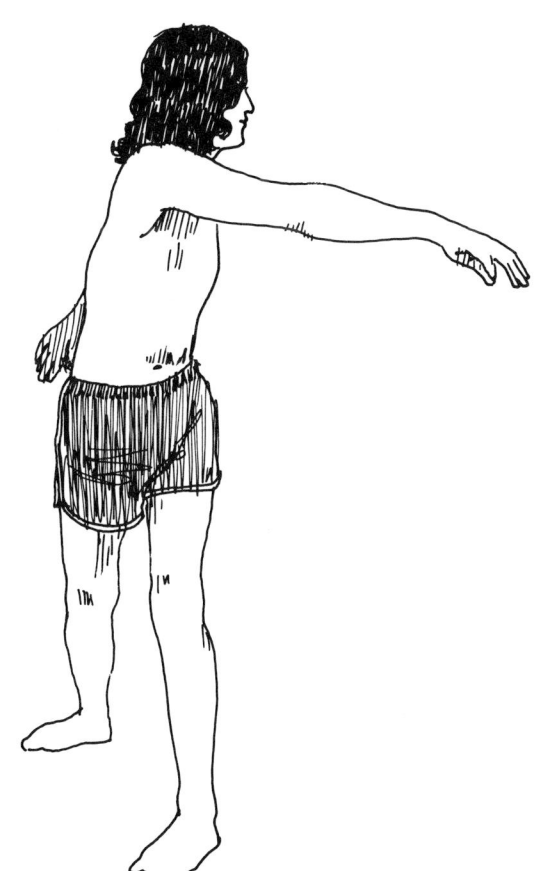

Airplane Swings

1. Stand with feet about 2-3 feet apart.

2. Bend forward from hips, upper body parallel to floor.

3. Swing arms vigorously from side to side. Turn head and torso to look at raised arm. Repeat 8-10 times. Exhale to each side.

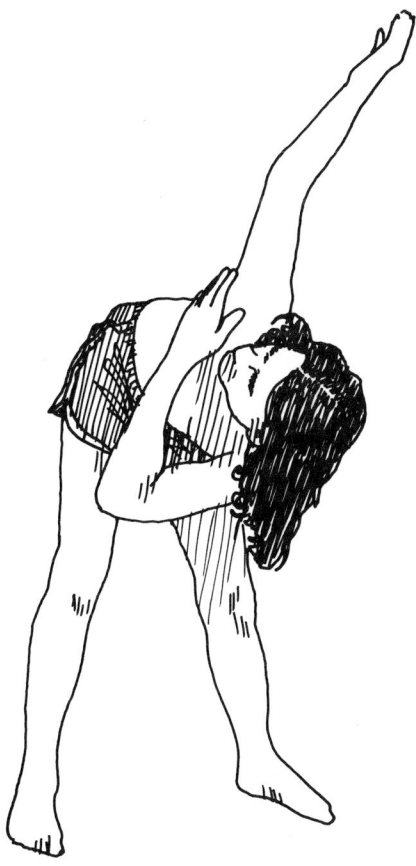

WARM-UPS

Brushing the Floor

1. Stand with feet hip-width apart.

2. As if holding buckets of paint in each hand, begin to swing your arms forward and up as you inhale; down and back as you exhale.

3. Bend knees so fingertips touch floor as you swing down. Straighten your legs when arms are up and back.

Standing Squats

1. Squat with hands on floor between your feet, elbows on the inside of your knees. Inhale.

2. Forcefully exhale as you straighten your legs into a standing forward bend, hands remaining on the floor.

3. Inhale and squat.

4. Repeat 8-10 times.

Trapeze

1. Sit with legs outstretched and together as in preparation for Paschimottanasana.

2. Raise arms forward as if to hold onto a trapeze bar. Extend your spine fully by lifting out of your pelvis.

3. Lower the trunk backward halfway to the floor, then lift back upright. Repeat 8-10 times.

4. Lower the trunk backward halfway to the floor, then down so lower back is on the floor. Lift halfway up. Repeat 8-10 times.

5. Relax.

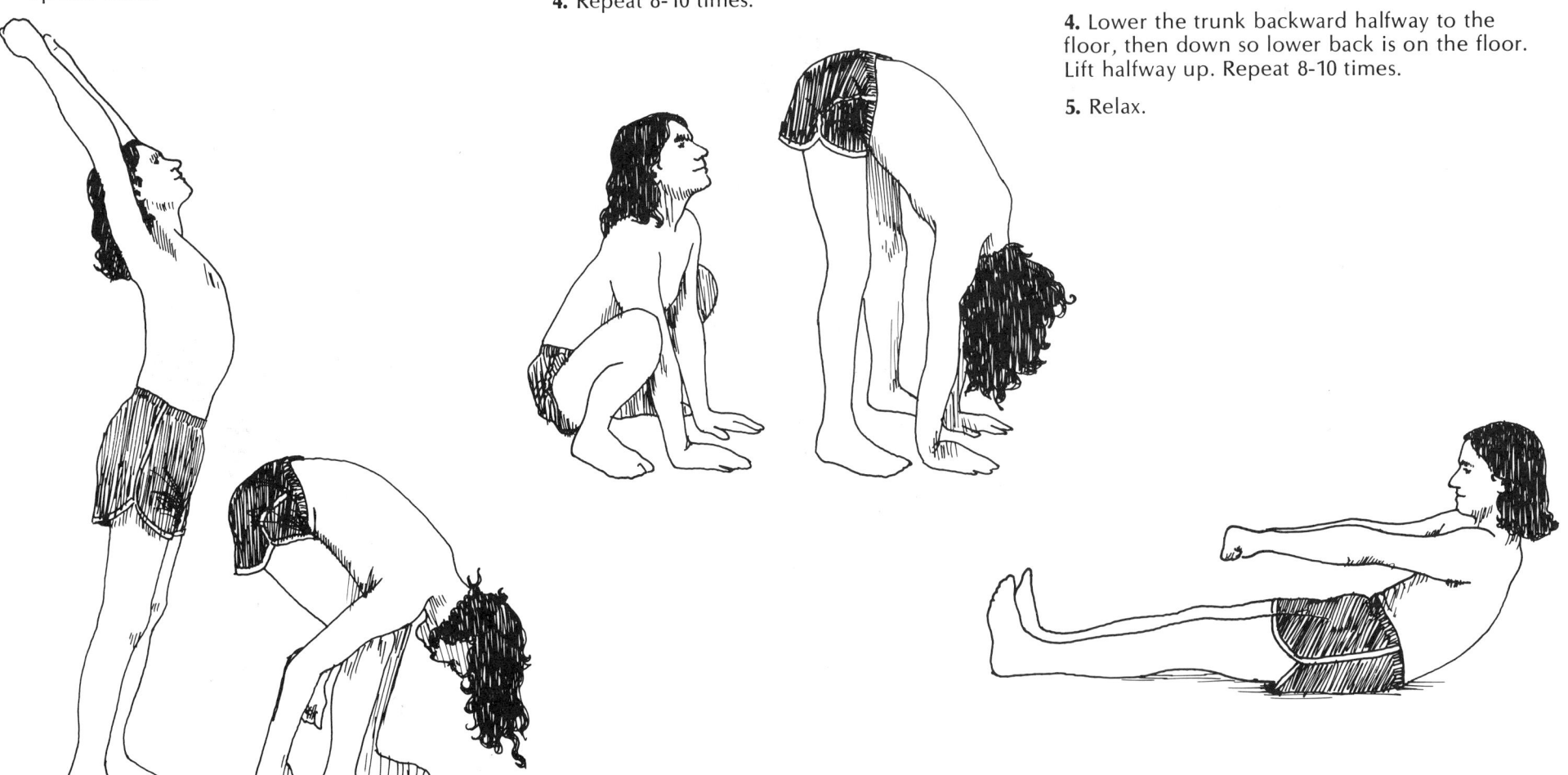

Sitting Airplane

1. Sit on buttocks with legs extended in front of you. Straighten legs and spread apart.

2. Stretch left hand to right foot as you forcefully exhale.

3. Inhale as you return to center.

4. Exhale forcefully as you stretch the right hand to the left foot.

5. Continue this side to side motion, vigorously swinging your arms 8-10 times.

Squatting

1. Stand erect with feet hip-width apart. Raise your arms in front of you, perpendicular to your body.

2. Keeping your feet flat on the floor, come into a squatting position.

3. Release by slowly raising to a standing position.

4. Repeat.

Spinal Rocking

1. Sit with knees drawn towards chest, feet flat on floor. Clasp hands around your knees.

2. Tuck chin toward chest and gently rock back on your rounded spine, stretching your legs overhead as you rock back.

3. Rock forward. Continue rocking to loosen muscles of your back.

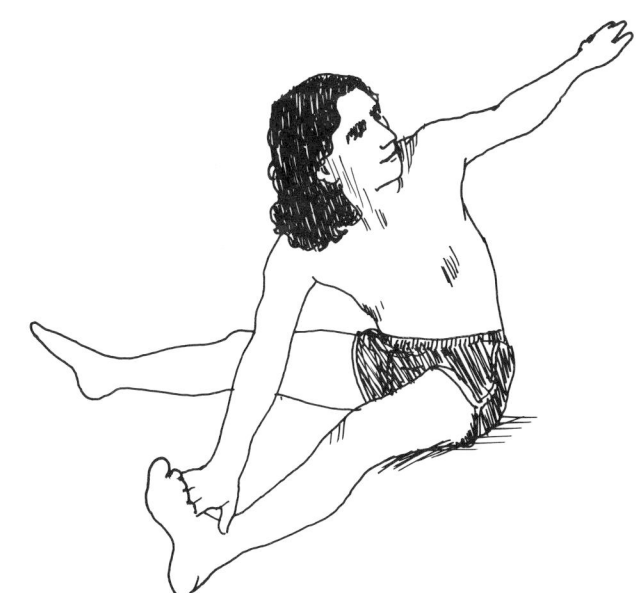
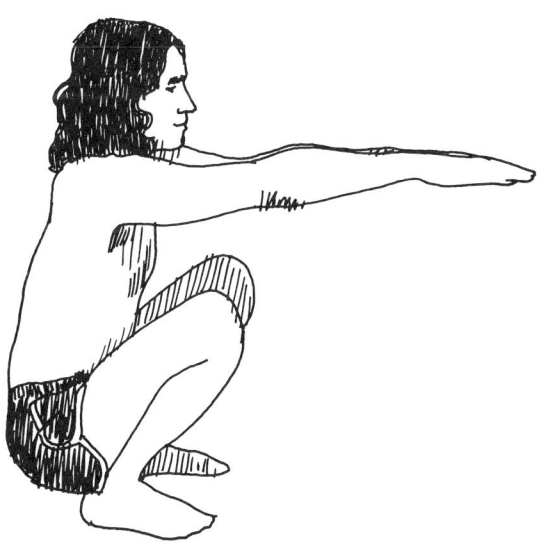
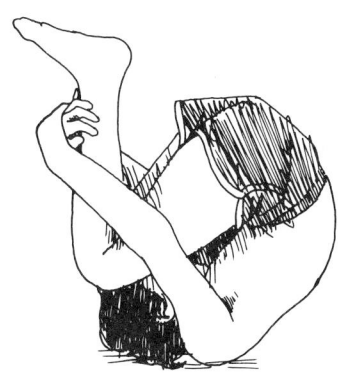

WARM-UPS

Full Torso Rotations

1. Stand, hands on waist.

2. Keeping the lower body stationary, slowly rotate the upper body about the waist, spine straight, in widening circles.

3. Reverse the rotation.

Downward-Facing Triangle

1. Sit on your heels, then bend forward, pushing your hands along the floor.

2. Raise your buttocks and straighten your arms and legs.

3. Press first one heel and then the other to the floor alternately, then press both at once.

4. Straighten the spine by pushing the sternum towards the floor and rotating the coccyx upwards. Kapalabhati.

Danda—Indian Push-ups

1. Come into Downward-Facing Triangle.

2. Lower knees, chest, and chin to the floor.

3. Slide forward between your arms, arching up and back, supported only by your hands and feet.

4. Repeat 1, 2, and 3 to exhaustion.

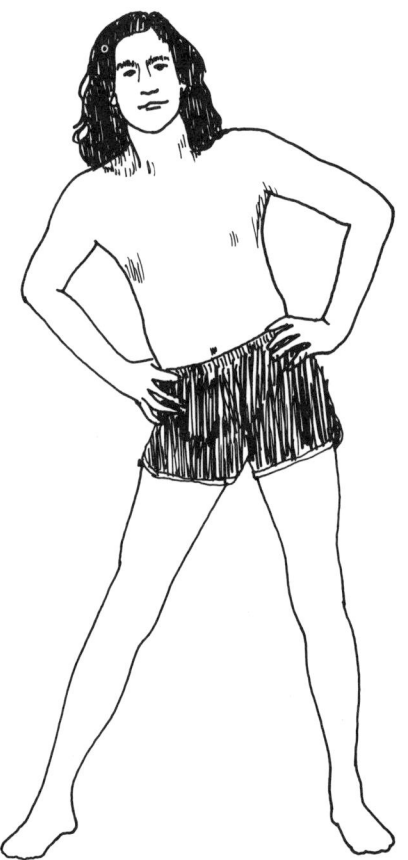

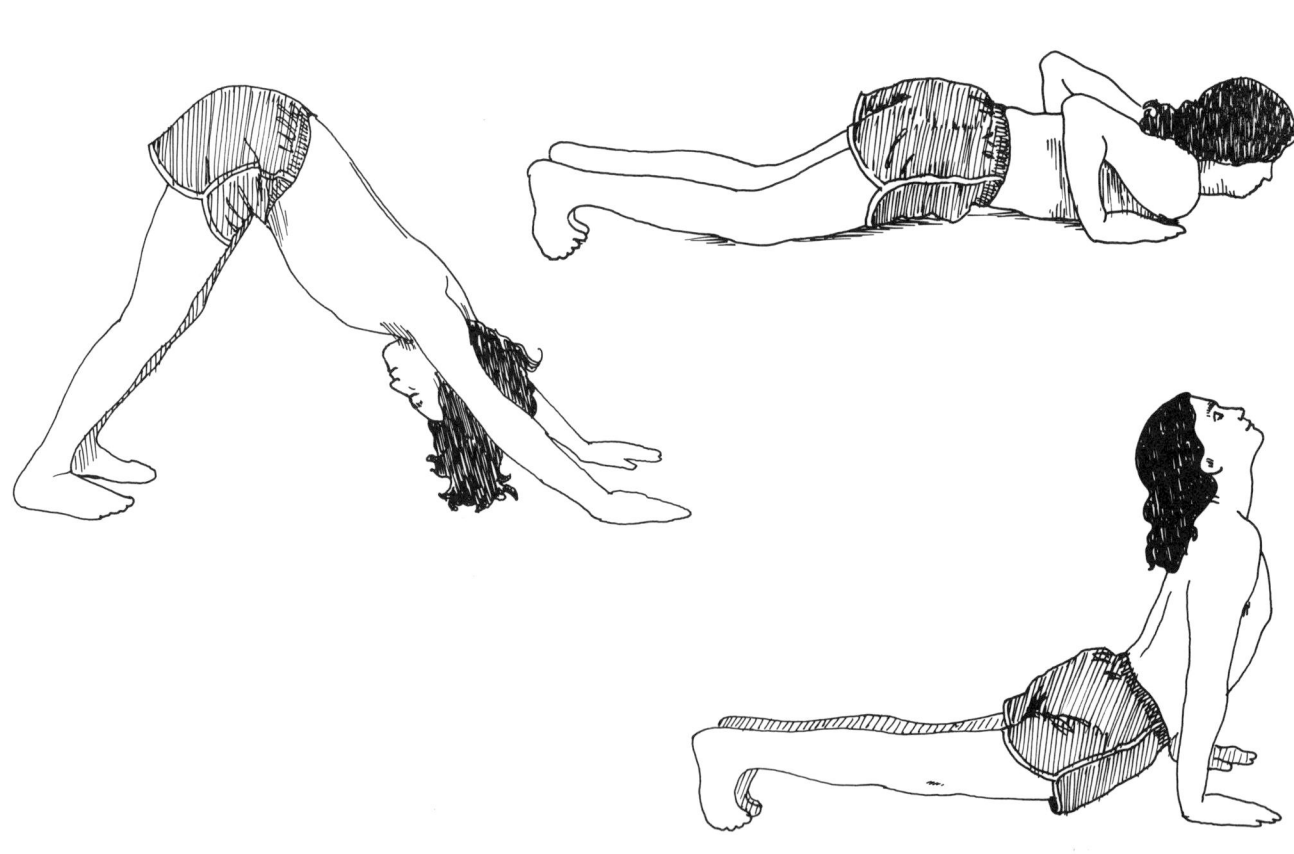

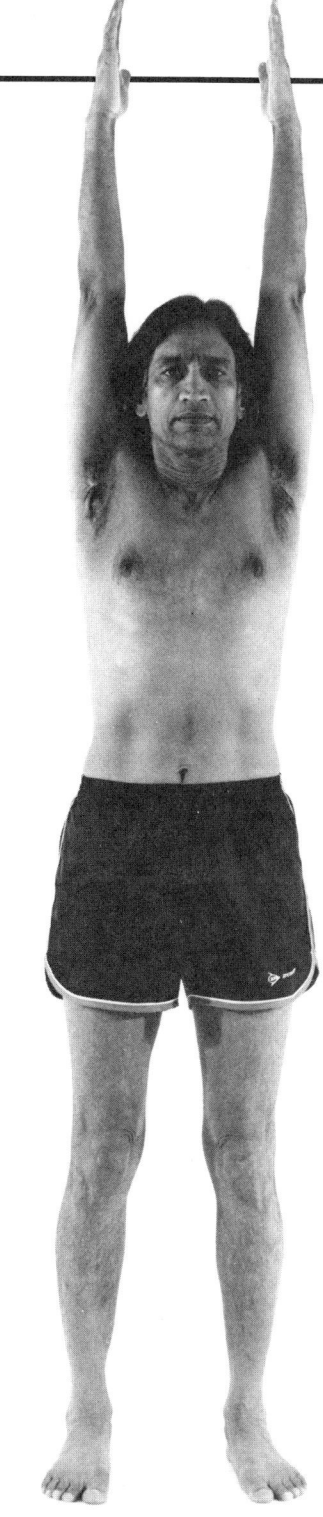

TADASANA—MOUNTAIN

Technique:

1. Stand erect with feet hip-width apart and parallel to one another so that both big toes point forward. Distribute your weight evenly on both feet and evenly between your heels and toes.

2. Lift up your kneecaps by tightening your thighs. Tuck your tailbone under, which will slightly contract your buttocks.

3. Lift your abdominal muscles and lengthen your lower back muscles.

4. Lift sternum. Breathe to fill your lungs completely—filling the space under your collarbones.
    Breathe normally

5. Lengthen the back of your neck by lifting your head up and out from your shoulders.

6. Raise your arms up overhead, stretching your arms from the armpit to the little-finger side of your hand. Palms face each other. Keep shoulders relaxed to leave space between your ears and shoulders.
    Inhale and lift

7. Softly focus your gaze at a point in front of you along the horizon. Hold.
    Breathe normally

Benefits of Tadasana:

1. Leaves you feeling grounded and balanced in both body and mind by bringing the body into proper and balanced alignment.

2. Provides the basic alignment for all other standing postures.

3. Helps correct postural deviations and their associated pain, which results from bearing body weight unevenly on your feet, standing with your weight on only one leg, or standing with one foot turned outwards.

Helpful Hints and Precautions:

The parallel placement of your feet may seem unusual at first. By learning to stand in this position, you will begin to experience a sense of balance and groundedness that comes when feet and body are aligned.

SURYA NAMASKAR—SUN SALUTATION

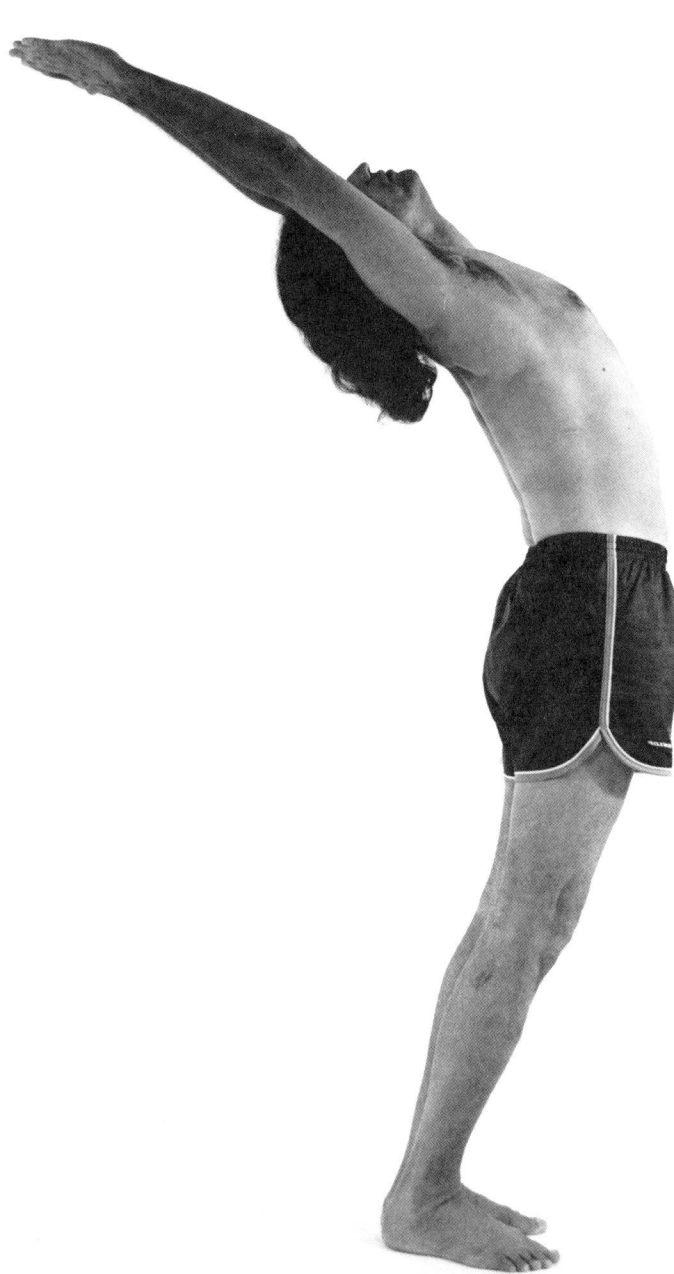

Technique:

1. Stand erect with your feet hip-width apart and parallel to one another. Join your palms in prayer position in front of your chest, with your elbows pointed downward.   **Exhale**

2. Slowly raise your arms over your head, releasing your hands. Keeping your head between your arms, palms facing each other, bend slightly backward.   **Inhale**

3. Bend forward from your hips. Place the palms of your hands on the floor beside your feet. Bend your knees if necessary.   **Exhale**

4. Stretch your right leg behind you. Rest your right knee on the floor and curl your toes under your feet. Your left foot is stationary between your hands, with your chest touching your left knee. Arch your back, open your chest and look up toward the ceiling. Hold.   **Hold in**

5. Straighten your right knee and bring your left leg back so that both feet and legs are together, toes under. Straighten your arms so that your body forms a straight incline, as in a push-up position.

6. Lower your knees, chest, and chin to the floor with your buttocks up in the air.   **Exhale**

7. Slide forward, lowering your hips and abdomen to the floor. Uncurl your toes, raise your head, neck, and chest into the Bhujangasana (Cobra) position. The lower part of your body remains on the floor.   **Inhale**

8. Curl your toes under once again. Raise your hips until your arms and legs are straight, forming a triangle with your body and the floor. Keep elbows straight, shoulders relaxed. Keep your head between your arms and your feet flat on the floor. Your back is straight.   **Exhale**

9. Take a long step forward, placing your right foot between your hands. Lower your left knee to the floor, raise your head to look toward the ceiling.   **Inhale**

10. Step forward with your left leg, bringing the left foot beside the right. Place your hands, palms down, beside your feet. Straighten your legs and bring your ribs and chest down along your legs.

11. Reach out with your arms and lift to standing position, stretching your arms straight overhead. Look at your fingers.   **Inhale**

12. Lower your arms back to prayer position in front of your chest and then down to your sides.   **Exhale**

13. Repeat the entire sequence leading with the left leg. This completes one round of the Sun Salutation.

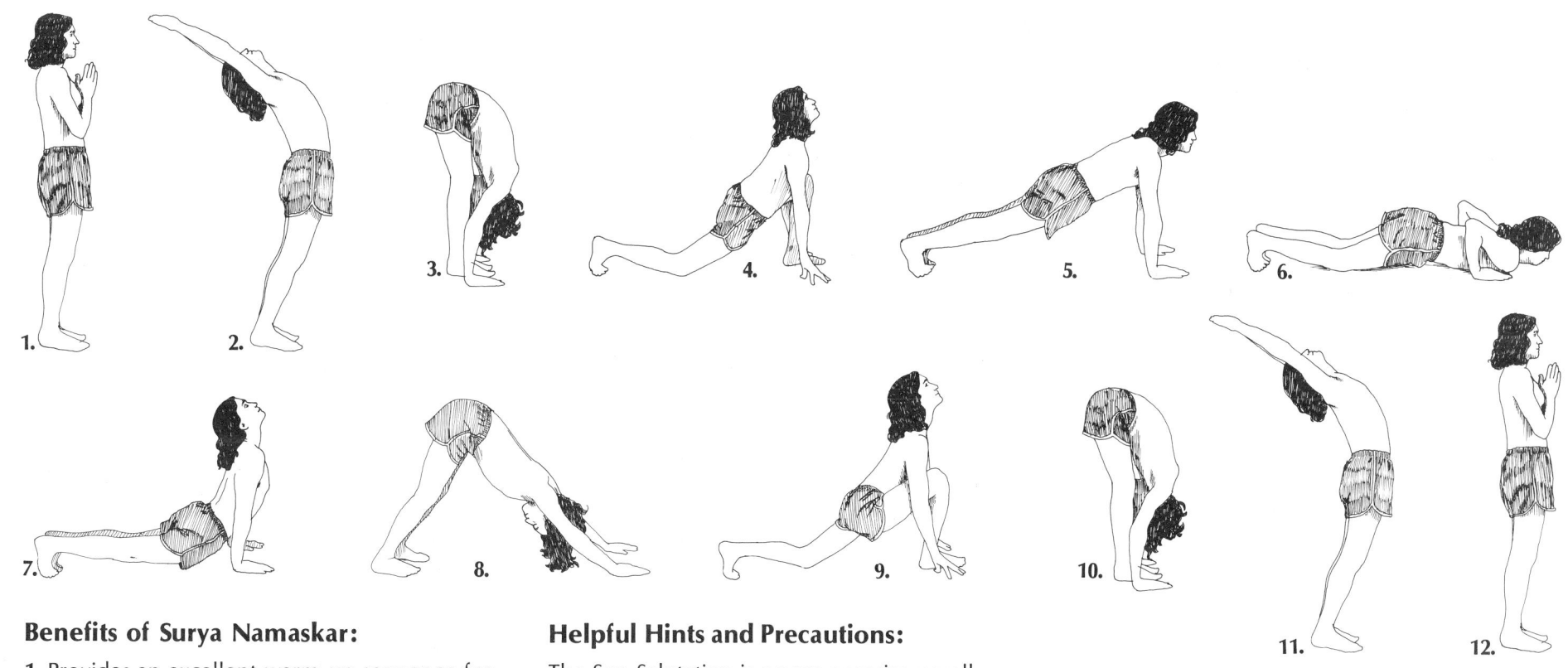

Benefits of Surya Namaskar:

1. Provides an excellent warm-up sequence for stretching, toning, and invigorating the whole body.

2. Tones the digestive system by alternately stretching and compressing the abdominal region. Massages the liver, stomach, spleen, intestines and kidneys. Activates the digestive processes and helps eliminate constipation and dyspepsia.

3. Thoroughly ventilates the lungs. Oxygenates the blood and removes carbon dioxide and toxic gases from the respiratory tract.

4. Stretches and massages the spinal column, toning the nervous system and regulating the functions of the sympathetic and parasympathetic nervous systems.

Helpful Hints and Precautions:

The Sun Salutation is a yoga exercise usually done before your other daily yoga exercises. It limbers the spine as well as all the muscles of the body, and invigorates the entire system. This exercise is traditionally practiced in the early morning as a salute to the sun. It is a combination of postures and breathing exercises that, when mastered, produces a flowing bodily movement.

In case of lower back stiffness, it is best to stretch the spine sideways (by performing Utthita Trikonasana—Triangle, for example) before doing the forward and backward bends that are parts of Surya Namaskar.

UTTHITA TRIKONASANA—TRIANGLE

Technique:

1. Stand with your feet 3 to 3½ feet apart. Turn your right foot out 90 degrees to the right. Turn your left foot slightly, about 30 degrees to the right. The right foot line should bisect the left. Keep your pelvis facing forward and your buttocks tilted under and forward.

2. Raise your arms sideways from your shoulders so that they are parallel to the floor.

Inhale deeply

3. Extend your upper body sideways to the right, extending from your hips. Push your hips to the left.

Exhale slowly

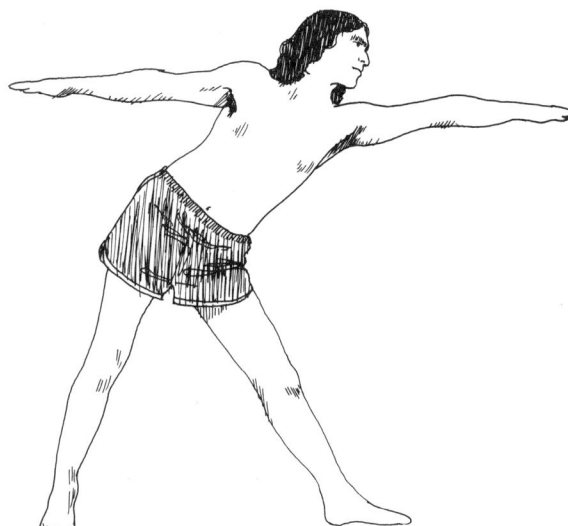

4. Lower your upper body, moving both arms simultaneously, the right one down, the left one up. If possible, rest your right palm on the floor next to your right foot. If this is difficult, lightly place your hand on your leg.

5. Raise your left arm toward the ceiling so it is in line with the right shoulder. Turn your head to gaze at your left hand. Hold.

Breathe deeply

6. Lift your upper body back to standing position by leading and lifting with your left arm.

Inhale

7. Repeat the posture to the left.

Benefits of Utthita Trikonasana:

1. Provides alternate flexing and relaxing of the body's lateral and dorsal muscles, bringing resilience to the spine and proper placement to the bones and muscles of the hips.

2. Tones the muscles of the legs.

3. Tones the nerves of the spine and aids digestion.

4. Provides relief from menstrual cramps.

Helpful Hints and Precautions:

As you do the Triangle, keep your tailbone tucked and pelvis facing forward for proper alignment and to protect your lower back from overstrain. In the beginning, you may find it helpful to do the Triangle while standing against a wall, in order to maintain proper alignment and balance.

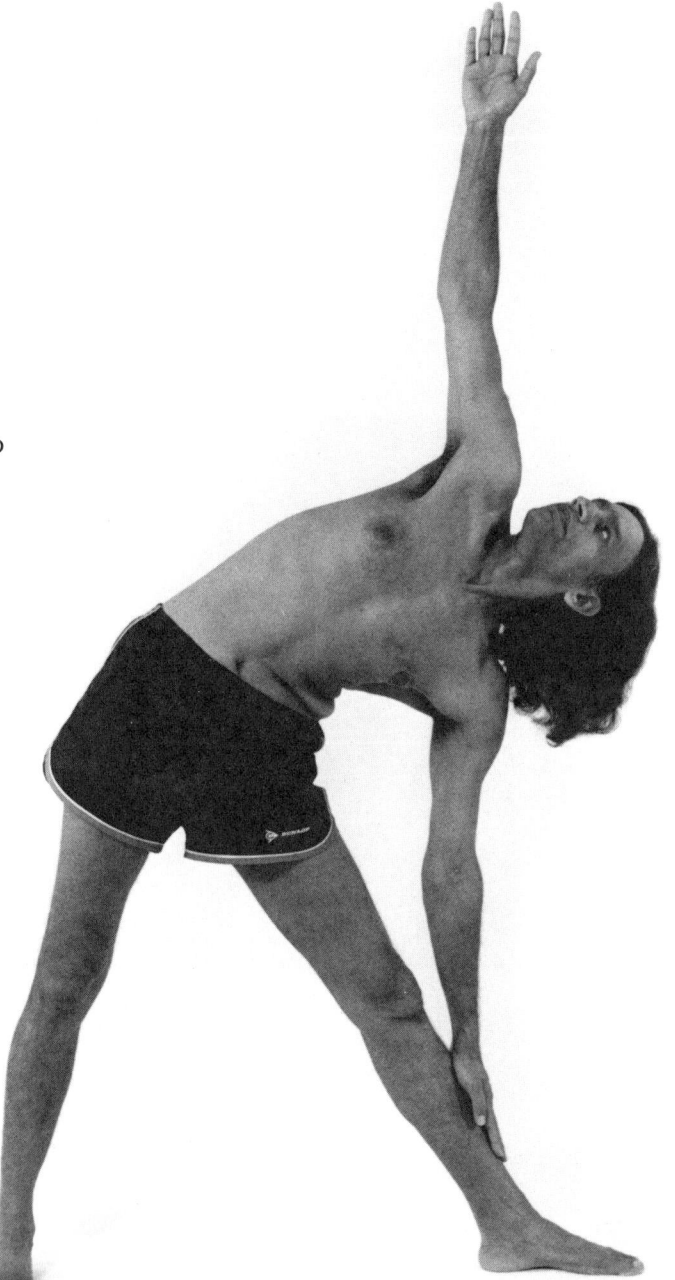

NAVASANA—BOAT

Technique:

1. Lie flat on your abdomen with your arms extended in front of you.

2. Simultaneously raise your legs straight behind you and your arms in front. Press your lower abdomen against the floor. Elongate your whole body. Keep the back of your neck lengthened as you tuck your chin slightly.

Inhale then exhale

3. Hold.

Breathe normally

4. Release, resting on the floor, turning your head to one side.

Exhale

5. Raise your legs straight behind you and your arms out from your shoulders, perpendicular to your body. Press your lower abdomen against the floor.

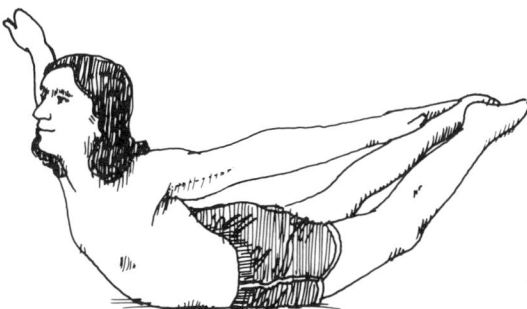

6. Hold.

Breathe normally

7. Relax.

Exhale down

8. Raise your legs straight behind you and your arms behind your back, interlacing your fingers. Press your lower abdomen against the floor.

Inhale then exhale

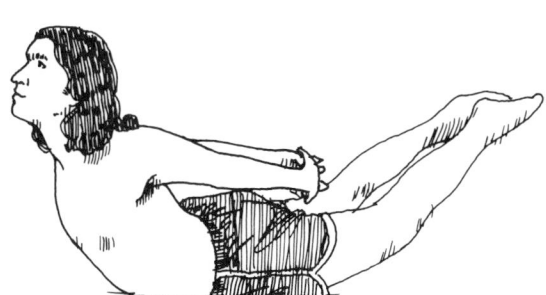

9. Hold.

Breathe normally

10. Release. Rest on the floor with your head turned to one side.

Exhale down

Breathe normally

Benefits of Navasana:

1. Strengthens the muscles of your back.

2. Trains your body to use the strength of the back muscles, rather than the arms, to lift into Bhujangasana (Cobra).

3. Provides kidneys with a fresh blood supply through the holding and releasing of the posture.

4. Energizes the entire body.

Helpful Hints and Precautions:

Practice this posture without strain and with consistency. If your back muscles are weak, proceed slowly, gradually increasing your holding time.

Navasana should not be practiced after the third month of pregnancy.

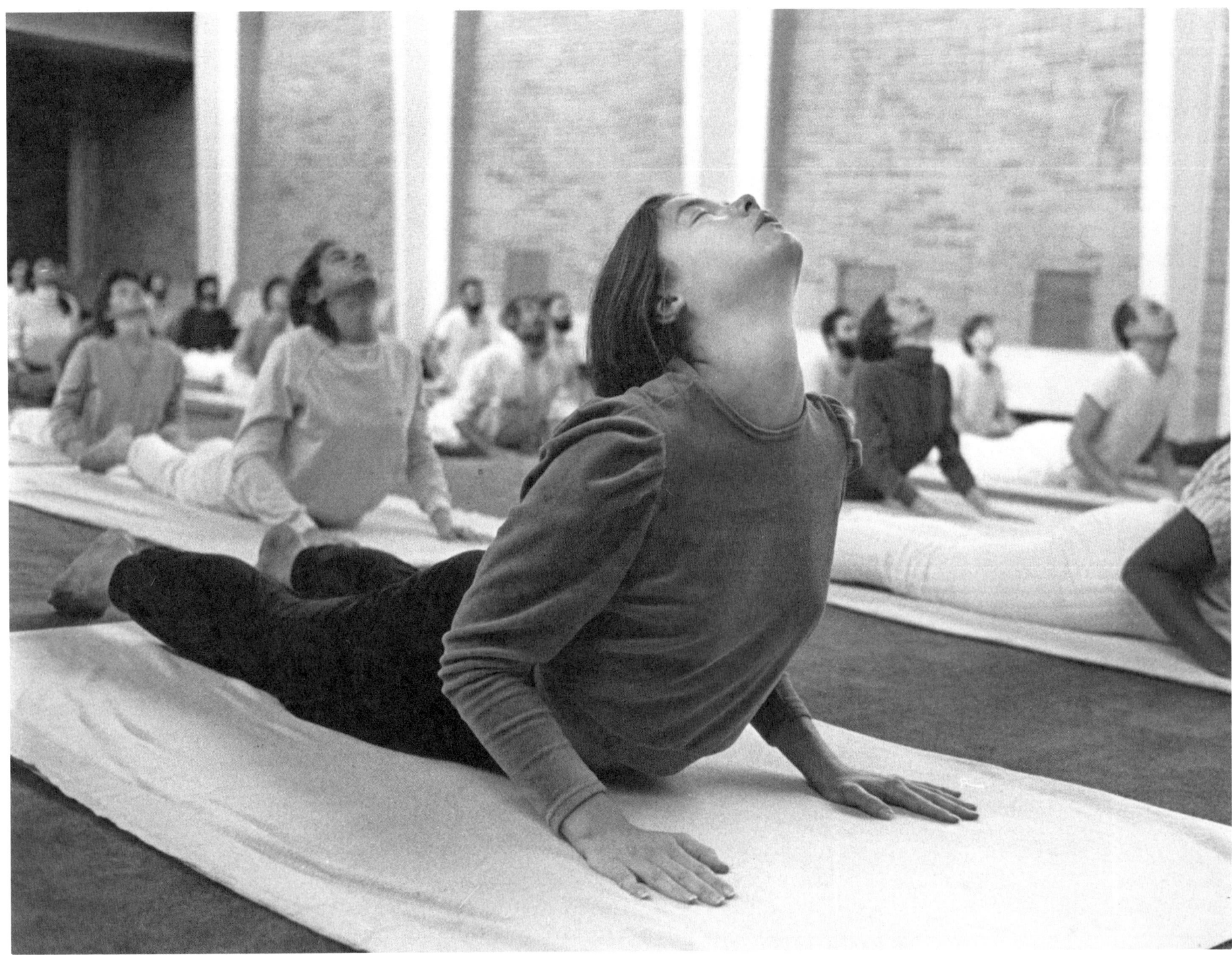

BHUJANGASANA—COBRA

Technique:

1. Lie on the floor, facing downwards with your forehead on the floor.

2. Extend your legs, feet together, kneecaps lifted, and toes pointed. Press your pubic bone against the floor.

3. Place palms beneath your shoulders, fingers pointed forward.

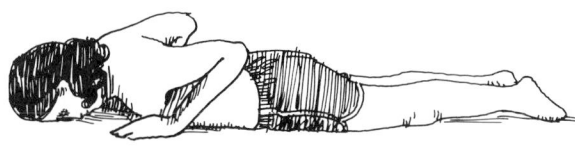

4. Begin raising your forehead, eyes, nose, chin, and throat from the floor, placing no weight on your hands.

Inhale slowly

5. Continue lifting your torso, as far as you can by using the strength of your back muscles.

Exhale

6. Placing weight on your hands, continue elongating your spine. For this purpose roll your eyes up and back, lift your sternum, open your chest, continue pressing your lower abdomen against the floor.

Breathe normally

7. Keep your elbows at your sides, slightly bent, your shoulders relaxed and low.

8. Hold the posture.

Kapalabhati 15 x

9. Using the strength of your back muscles again, slowly lower your abdomen, then your chest, neck, chin, nose, and forehead back to rest on the floor.

Exhale slowly

10. Bring your arms back to your sides. Turn your head to rest on one side of your face.

11. Relax.

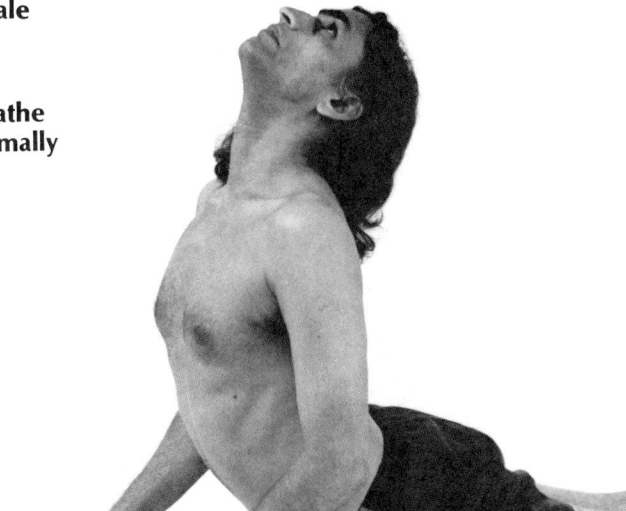

Benefits of Bhujangasana:

1. Tones and strengthens the spinal region.

2. Lessens rigidity in the chest through expansion.

3. Draws increased blood supply to the spinal cord, strengthening the nervous system.

4. Massages the abdominal organs.

5. Relieves constipation through stretching of the abdomen.

6. Relieves after-meal flatulence.

7. Normalizes thyroid gland.

8. During the holding, forces old blood from the kidneys. During the return position, provides a fresh supply of blood to the kidneys, giving this position a diuretic effect.

9. Brings about a sense of security and self-confidence because of the upright carriage.

10. Strengthens the reproductive system.

Helpful Hints and Precautions:

As with all yoga postures, sudden or jerking movements may cause stiffness. Train your body gently through consistent practice rather than by forcing it. You should rise up to the Cobra position using only the muscles of your back, not your arms. You may want to place your palms on the back of your thighs and rise up with no support.

The Cobra should not be done after the third month of pregnancy.

DHANURASANA—BOW

Technique:

1. Lie flat on your stomach, with arms along your sides. Relax your back. Grasp your ankles with your hands (grasp one at a time if easier). Place your knees, ankles, and feet parallel and not any further apart than your hips, for correct postural alignment.

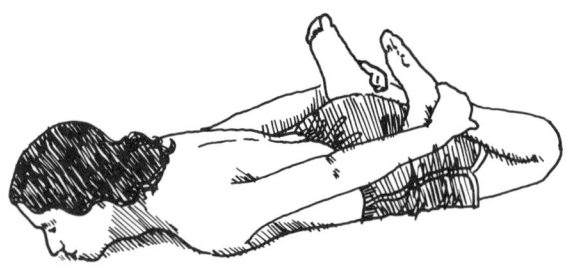

2. Simultaneously lift your head and, with a powerful contraction of buttocks and thighs, aided by your arms and hands, raise and extend your legs, aiming to align your knees with your shoulders. **Exhale**

3. Begin a rocking movement. Let the breath alone rock you. Rock 4-12 times. Let yourself be so unlimited in the rocking that the movement brings you back and forth, down onto your thighs and up onto your shoulder or clavicle area.

4. Hold the posture for 30-60 seconds. Squeeze the area between your shoulder blades, lifting the sternum. Continue contracting your buttocks. Rest neither on your ribs, nor on your lower abdomen, but on your middle abdomen. In order to tauten the Bow, use your hands to pull up your legs, and your feet to pull up your arms. **Breathe normally**

5. Lift still higher. **Kapalabhati**

6. Slowly lower your legs, release your hands, and unbend your legs. **Exhale**

7. Relax in Garbhasana (the Child Pose) in order to give a counter-stretch to your back.

Benefits of Dhanurasana:

1. Massages abdominal organs and muscles. Stimulates digestion and peristalsis.

2. Massages and stimulates the solar plexus (the complex of nerves in the pit of the stomach).

3. Through the powerful stretch to the abdomen helps the performance of Uddiyana Bandha (page II-55).

4. Activates the nerves of the spine by the intense backbending.

5. Activates the thyroid by stretching the front of the neck.

6. Improves peristalsis.

7. Irrigates kidneys with fresh blood supply, helping them to eliminate toxins.

8. Revitalizes the entire endocrine system, especially the pancreas, thyroid and gonads (recommended for cases of slow development in children, and underactive thyroid and obesity).

9. Helps relieve menstrual disorders as well as the back and abdominal pain that can accompany menopause.

Helpful Hints and Precautions:

The Bow should not be practiced by those suffering from hyperfunction of the thyroid or excessive growth of any other ductless glands. Do not perform the Bow after the third month of pregnancy. To avoid cramps in the feet, turn them towards your shins.

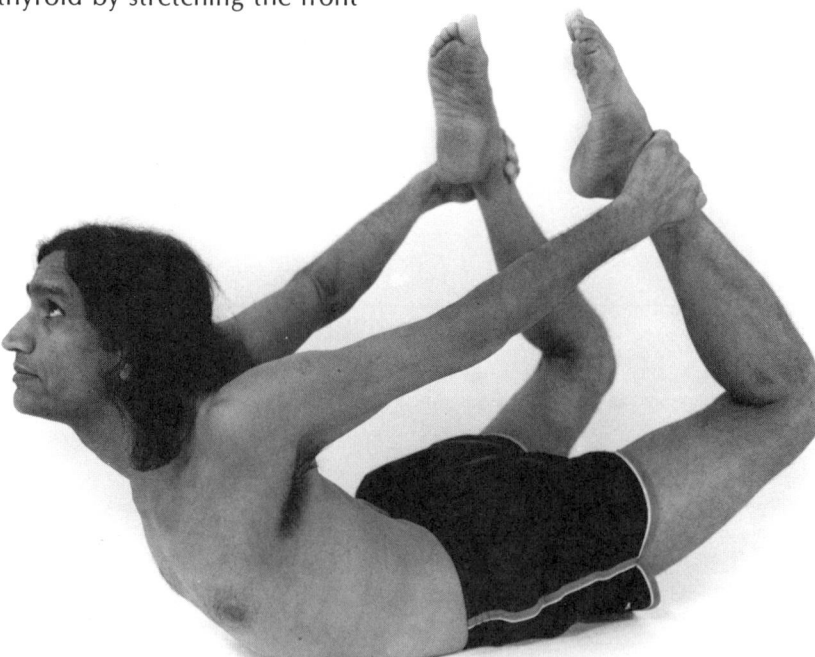

GARBHASANA—CHILD POSE

Technique:

1. Kneel on the floor with your knees and feet together, and your buttocks on your heels. Place your hands on your knees.

Ujjayi

2. Bending from your hips, lay your upper body down over your knees. Let your arms rest beside you with your hands next to your feet, palms facing upward; or extend your arms out in front of you.

Exhale

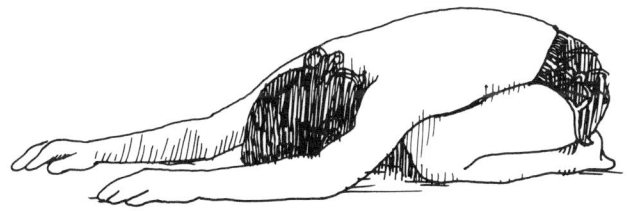

3. Raise your upper body back up to sitting.

Inhale

4. Relax.

Breathe normally

Benefits of Garbhasana:

1. Fully relaxes your back and spine, providing a good counterpose to any back-bending posture.

2. By relaxing in the position, leaves you with a feeling of security and nurturance.

Helpful Hints and Precautions:

If there is a gap between your buttocks and your heels, place a cushion or a folded blanket over your calves so that you bridge the gap and can sit in a relaxed way, which is the purpose of the posture.

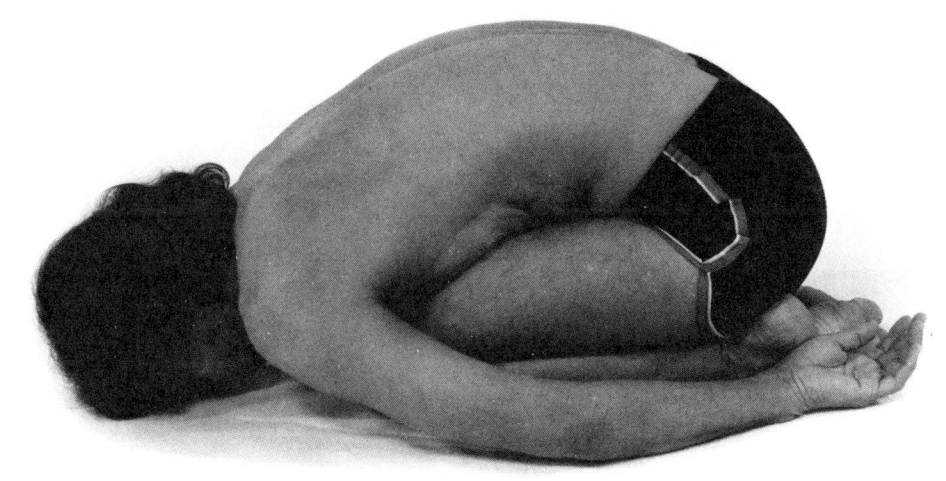

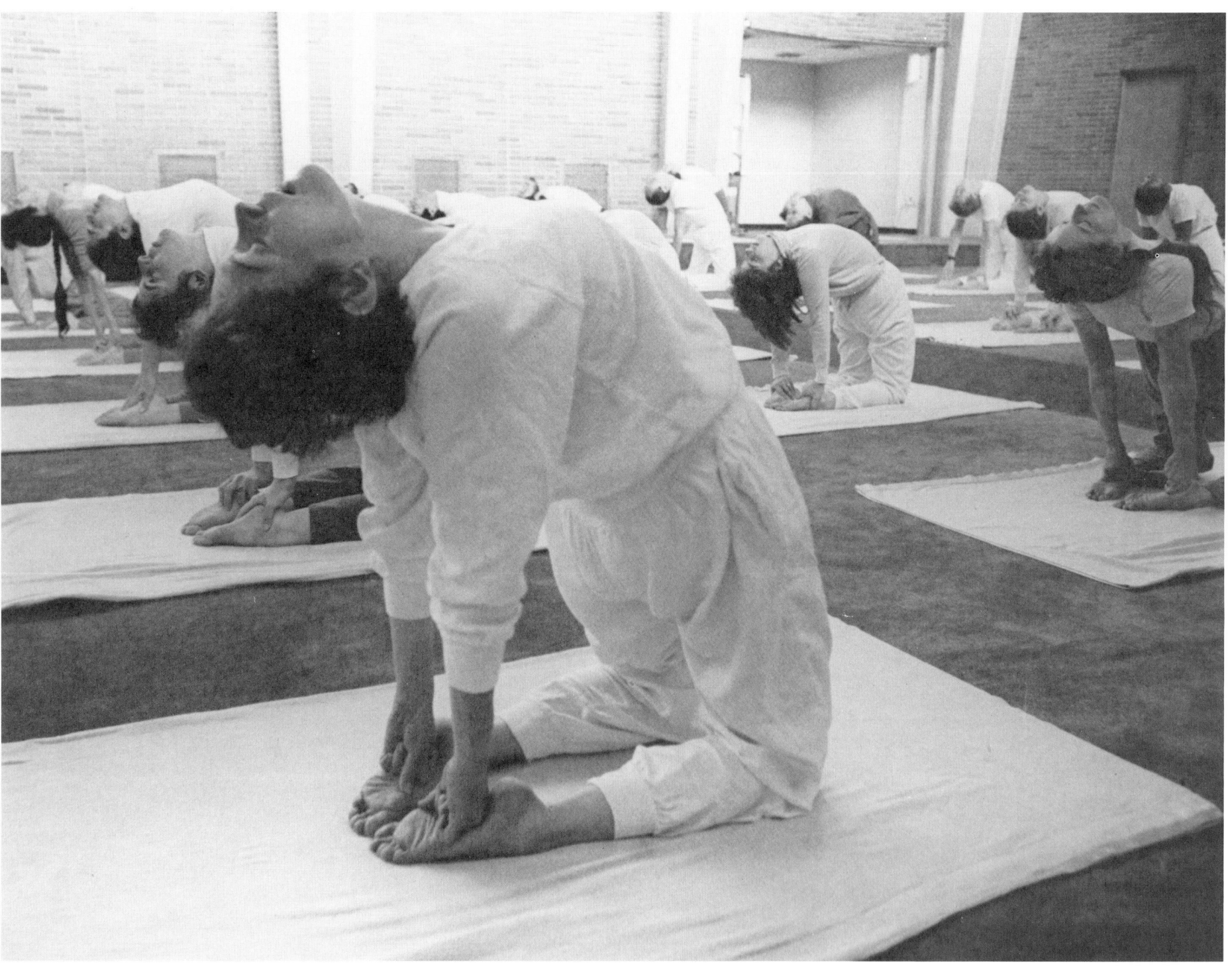

USHTRASANA—CAMEL

Technique:

1. Kneel comfortably with your hips resting on your heels. Place your hands on your knees.

2. Place your hands on the floor directly behind your feet or on the soles of your feet, with your fingers pointing away from your body.
Inhale

3. Drop your shoulders and head back. Shift your weight onto your arms.
Exhale

4. Lift your hips by pressing your pubic bone forward and stretching your thighs. Lift your sternum toward the ceiling and expand your ribs.
Inhale and lift

5. Hold and continue to press your pelvis forward. Keep your thighs perpendicular to the floor.
Breathe deeply

6. Release the position by lowering your hips to your heels. Keep your hands on the floor and your head back.
Exhale

7. Raise your head and shoulders.
Inhale

8. Return your hands to your knees and relax.
Exhale

Benefits of Ushtrasana:

1. Helps correct curving of upper back and drooping of shoulders.

2. Stretches and tones spine in its entirety.

3. Activates your abdominal organs through stretching.

4. Activates your kidneys through contraction.

Helpful Hints and Precautions:

As back stretching is difficult for many people, proceed slowly. The following approach will help you stretch your spine: lift your buttocks off your heels, curl your toes under, place your palms on your buttocks and glide them along the back of your legs, bringing them onto your heels or soles. Proceed then as in 4 and 5. To return, retrace the same path along the legs in the opposite direction. Avoid tensing your muscles as this will inhibit both flexibility and gradual, graceful movement.

If you are suffering from a hernia, do not practice Ushtrasana, the Camel.

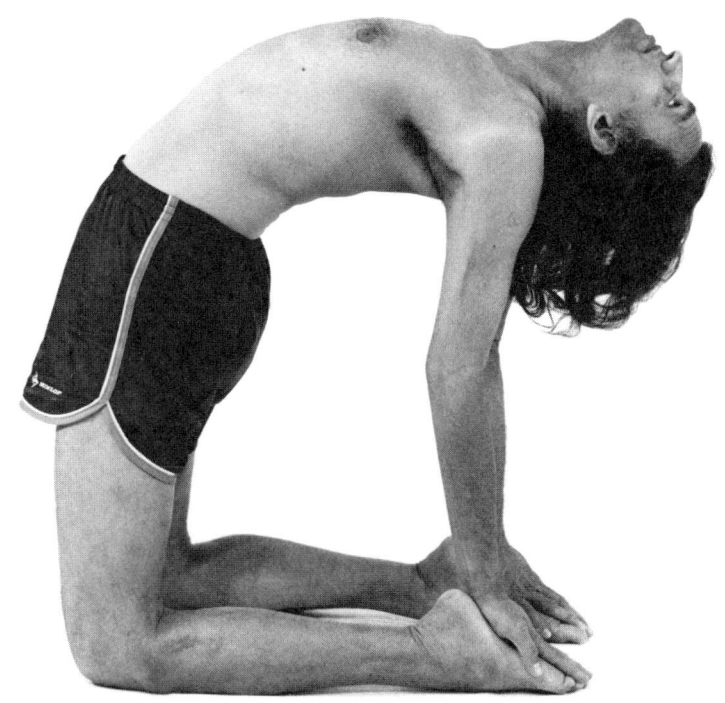

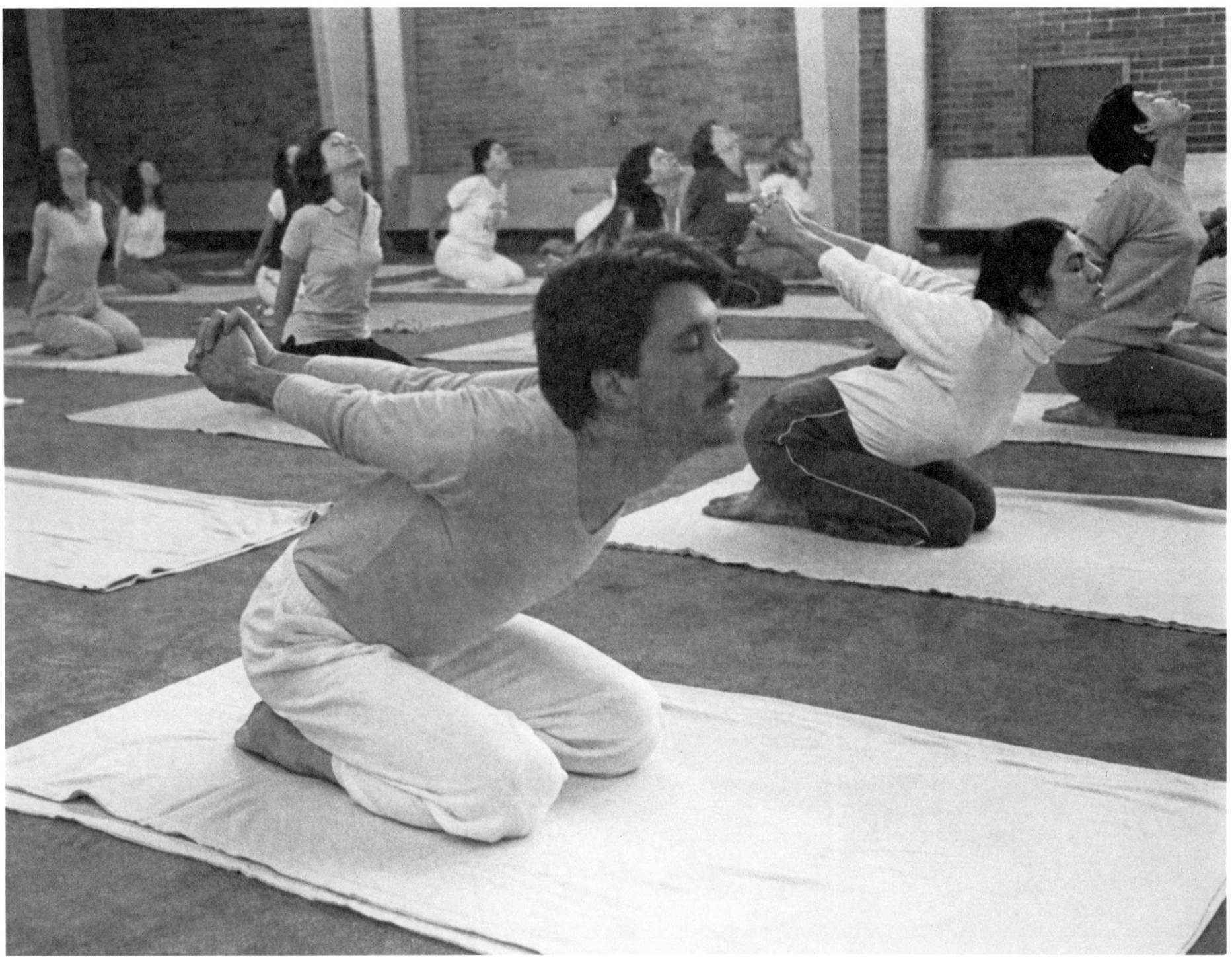

YOGA MUDRA—SYMBOL OF YOGA

Technique:

1. Sit on your heels. Place your hands on your knees.

2. Bring your arms behind you and interlace your fingers. Squeeze your shoulder blades together and open your chest.

Inhale deeply

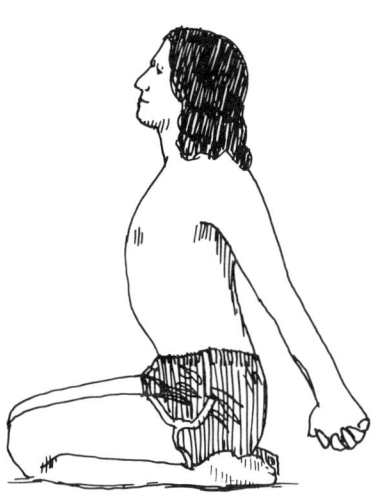

3. Simultaneously stretch your arms toward the ceiling and slowly bend forward from your hip joints, keeping the spine straight, the sternum lifted. Rest your forehead on the floor.

Exhale

4. Hold the position.

Breathe normally

5. Gradually return to sitting, elongating your spine.

Inhale slowly

6. Return your hands to your knees, and relax with eyes closed.

Exhale

Benefits of Yoga Mudra:

1. Helps restore abdominal organs to natural postion in abdominal cavity. (Organs often slip out of position due to poor digestion, poor intestine and colon activity.)

2. Provides external and internal pressure to the abdominal organs and muscles.

3. Creates an inner environment of humility and dissolution of false pride through the act of bowing. (Done with consciousness, this posture can help drive pride from us, as we bow humbly before our inner divinity, surrendering the ego part of our being).

4. Strengthens the nerves and muscles of the abdominal and pelvic areas.

Helpful Hints and Precautions:

For more of a stretch you can also invert your palms toward the ceiling.

If you suffer from chronic constipation, practice this posture gently, releasing it slowly and avoiding jerky movements.

Do not practice the Yoga Mudra if you have high blood pressure.

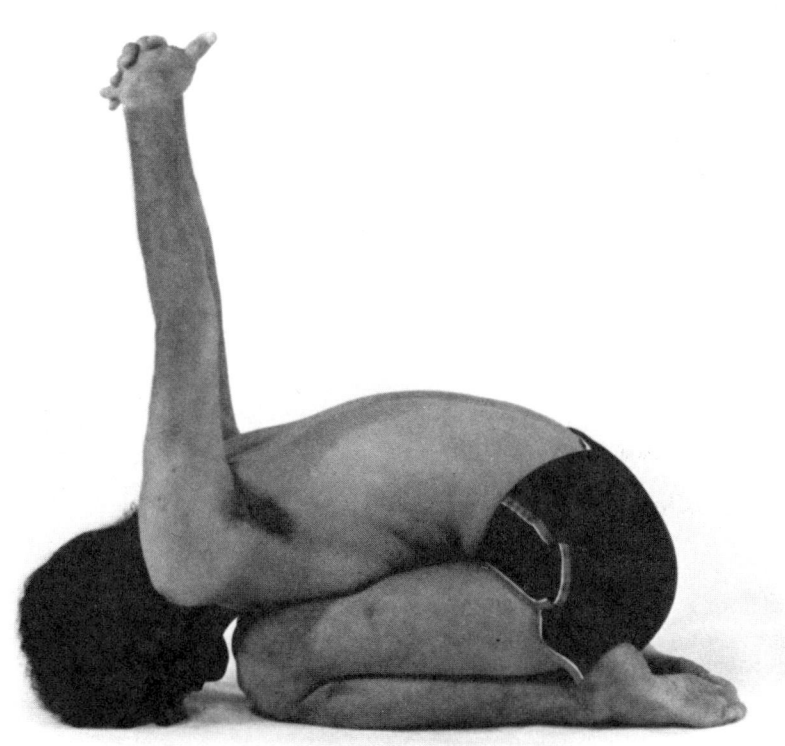

MAYURASANA—PEACOCK

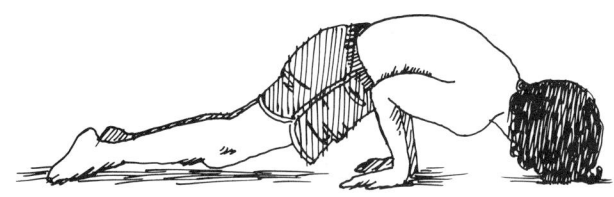

Technique:

1. Sit back on your heels with your knees apart.

2. Place palms on the floor with either (a) fingers pointing backwards towards feet, little fingers touching, or (b) insides of wrists touching with fingers pointing to the sides.

3. Press elbows and forearms together.   **Inhale**

4. Allow elbows to press into your diaphragm area (below ribs) as you bend forward, placing the top of your head on the floor. Be sure to keep your elbows together and pressed into your diaphragm or upper abdomen, not into the ribs.   **Exhale**

5. Stretch your legs back one leg at a time, keeping knees off the floor and feet together (weight is on toes, hands, and head).

6. Lift the head.

7. Gently come forward on the arms, leaning onto your elbows, lifting your toes up, and balancing on your hands. Legs remain straight.   **Inhale**

8. Hold this posture 30-60 seconds.   **Breathe normally**

9. Lower your head, then legs, then arms to the floor, finally coming back to sit on the heels with hands resting comfortably by your side.   **Exhale**

Benefits of Mayurasana:

1. Because elbows are pressed into the diaphragm and abdominal aorta, circulation is increased to all the abdominal organs after the release of the posture.

2. Breaks up toxic abdominal accumulations.

3. Improves digestion.

4. Strengthens upper body, chest, arms, and shoulders.

5. Increases concentration.

Helpful Hints and Precautions:

If doing this posture in Padmasana (the Lotus), the technique is the same, except that in Step 1 the legs are placed in Lotus postion. In Step 5, crossed legs are lifted behind you. Step 7 is skipped. Step 8: Balance 30 seconds with one crossed leg on top, then reverse so other crossed leg is on top for 30 seconds. (Whatever the holding time, allow it to be equal with each leg on top.)

Do not do this posture if you have had recent abdominal surgery or if you have a hernia.

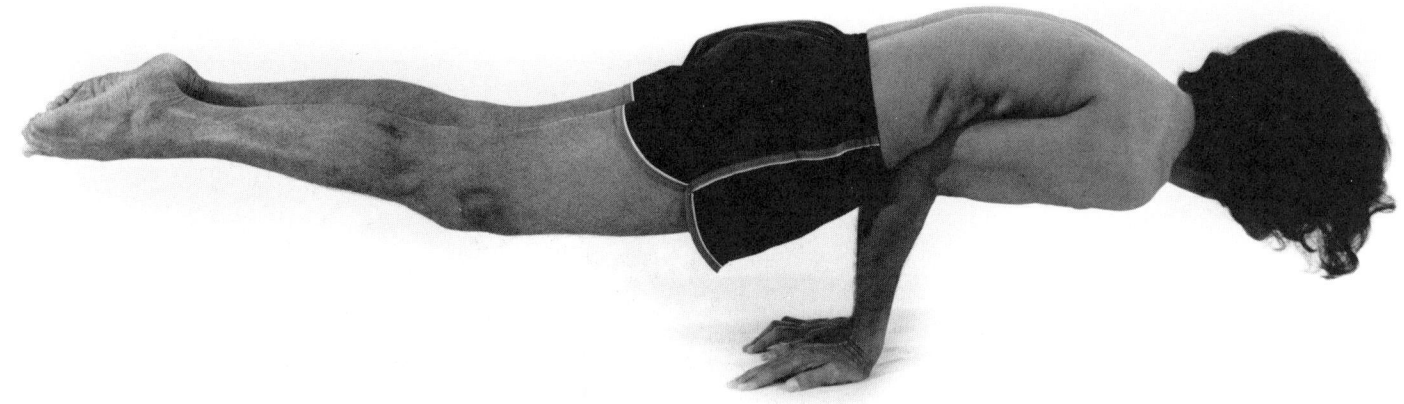

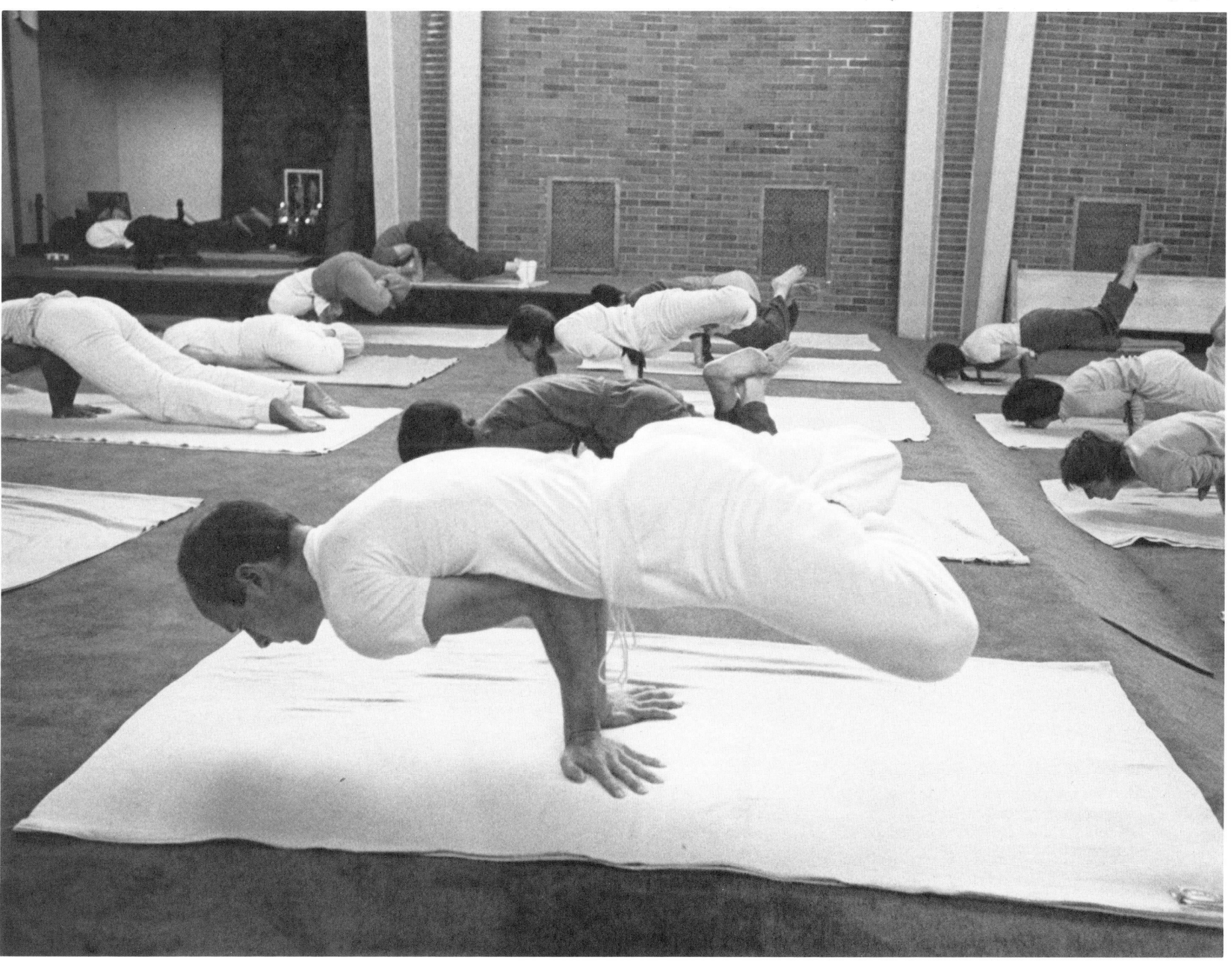

BHUNAMAN VAJRASANA—ABDOMINAL MASSAGE

Technique:

1. Kneel with your knees and feet together and buttocks resting on your heels.

2. Fold your arms in front of you and grasp both elbows. Press the right elbow against your abdomen on the right side beneath the rib cage.

Benefits of Bhunaman Vajrasana:

1. Gives a deep massage to your abdominal organs and muscles.

2. Through the deep massage beginning with the right elbow pressing into the abdomen, stimulates and balances digestion and peristalsis.

Helpful Hints and Precautions:

It is best not to do this posture on a full stomach. If your flexibility does not allow you to kneel comfortably with your buttocks on your heels, place a pillow between your buttocks and your feet. This will allow you to relax fully into the deep abdominal massage.

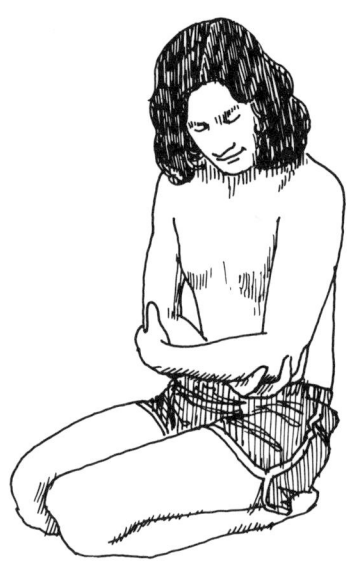

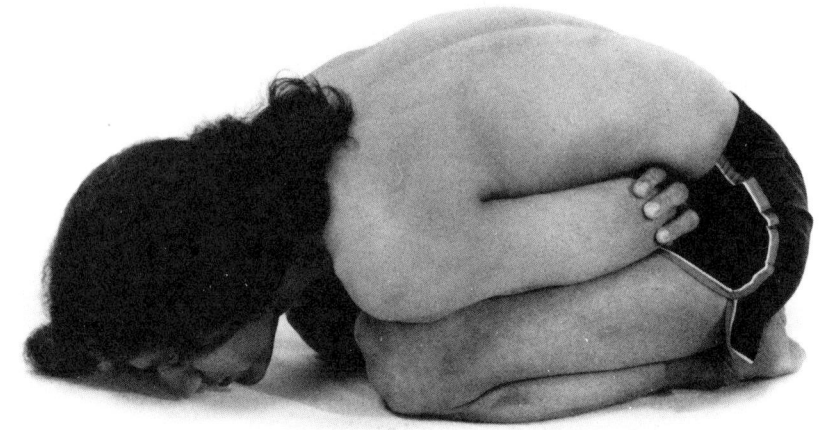

3. Bend forward from your hips, resting your upper torso across your thighs and your forehead on the floor.   **Exhale**

4. Relax, and allow your breath to be long and deep and your shoulders relaxed so that your arms may sink deep into your abdomen.   **Breathe normally**

5. Return to the upright position.   **Inhale up**

6. Reverse the position of your arms and repeat Steps 1-5.

ARDHA SHALABASANA—HALF LOCUST

Technique:

1. Lie flat, face downwards, legs extended, ankles together and toes pointed.

2. Place your arms either (a) at your sides with palms flat on the floor, or (b) under your body, with clenched fists placed in groin or thigh region. Keep entire length of arms touching floor.

3. Place your chin on the floor. Walk it as far forward as possible, stretching the front of the neck. — **Inhale deeply**

4. Raise the right leg, while leaning on the right side of the body. Keep the left side passive, left knee remaining on the floor. Concentration is on the stretch, not the lift. — **Exhale**

5. Lower the right leg. — **Hold breath out**

6. Take a deep breath in and out. — **Inhale then exhale**

— **Breathe normally**

7. Repeat Steps 4-6 raising your left leg and keeping your right side passive.

8. Rest until heartbeat normalizes.

Benefits of Ardha Shalabasana:

1. Draws blood to the sacral region of the spine through powerful contractions to the lumbar muscles.

2. Stimulates vagus nerve in the neck through contraction.

3. Through strengthening of the lumbar muscles, decreases chances of lower-back injury.

4. Recharges nervous system through increased blood flow to spinal column.

5. Through the spinal stretch, massages, tones and stimulates the entire digestive system. Stimulates peristalsis.

6. Provides a deep flushing of the kidneys through lower back contractions.

7. Raising of legs forces excess venous blood from them, helping to prevent varicosity.

Helpful Hints and Precautions:

Avoid bending either leg during the entire sequence. Avoid tilting your pelvis, and avoid tensing your calves. Contract the lower-back muscles so these muscles and the underlying kidneys receive a plentiful supply of blood when the posture is released.

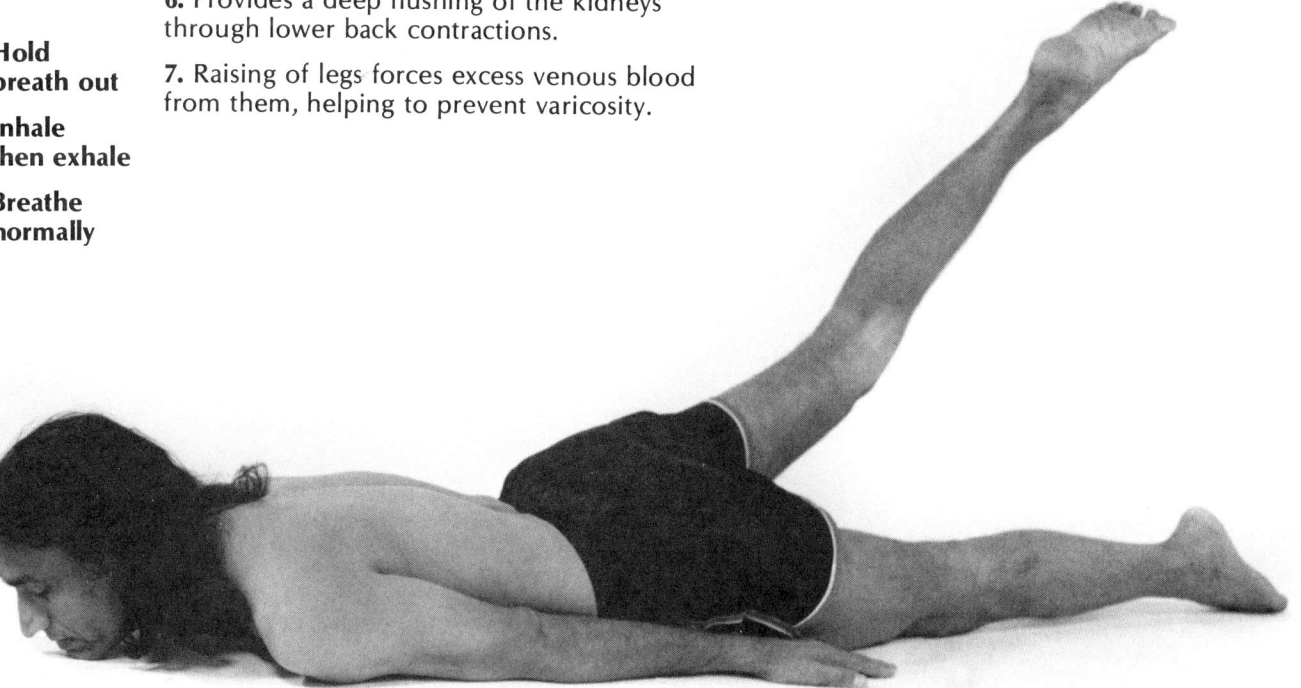

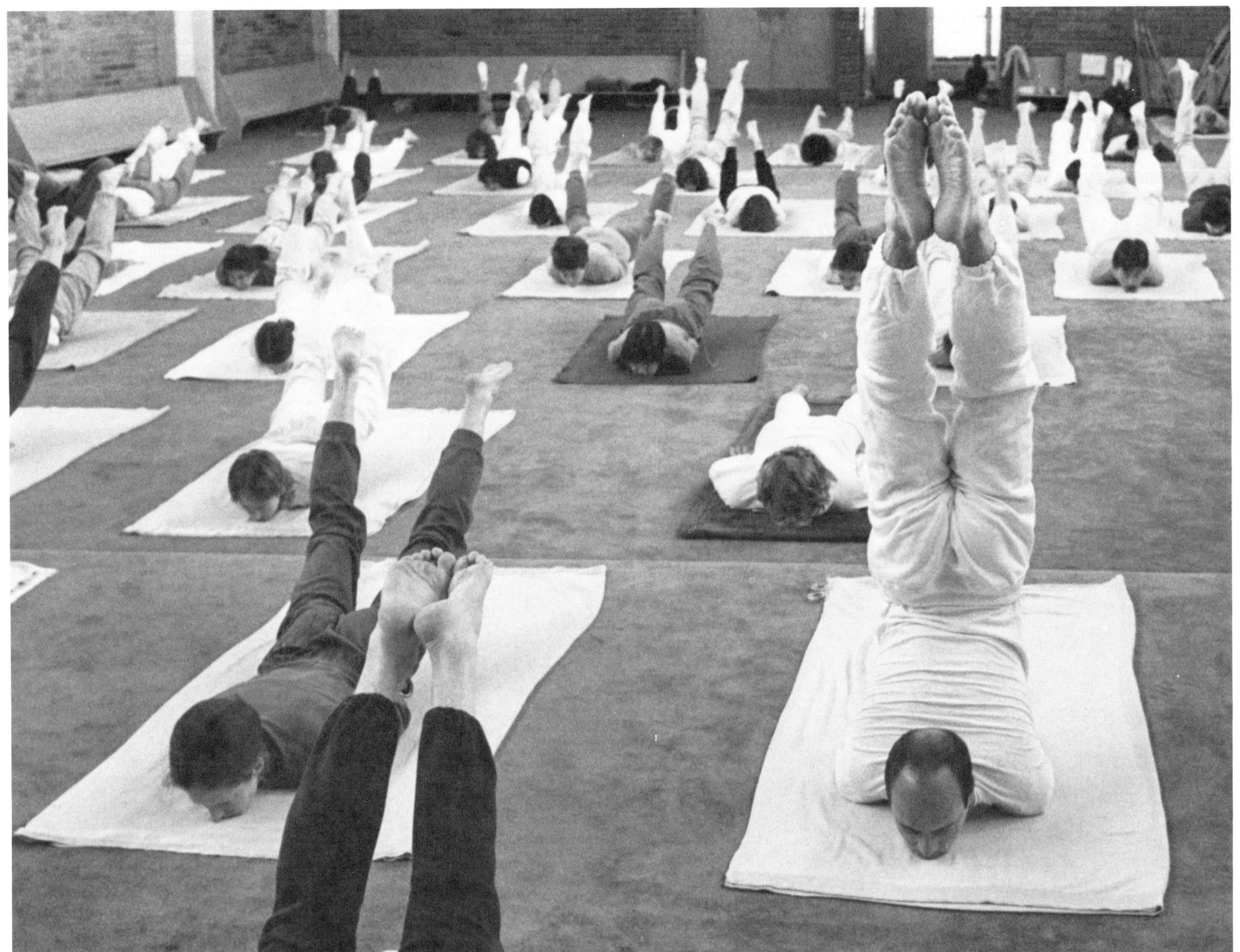

SHALABASANA—LOCUST

Technique:

1. Use the same starting position as Ardha Shalabasana (Half Locust). Clench fists into the groin area to provide more strength in the posture. Keep the entire length of your arms on the floor, elbows close together.

2. Through the power of a strong contraction of the muscles in the small of the back, raise both legs simultaneously.

Inhale, exhale up

3. Hold.

Hold breath out

4. Continue holding 30-60 seconds longer, placing the weight of your body towards your abdomen and chest.

Inhale when necessary

5. Lower your legs to the floor, placing your arms at your sides, turning your face to one side.

Exhale

6. Relax until breath and heart normalize.

Benefits of Shalabasana:

1. Similar to Ardha Shalabasana (Half Locust), yet more pronounced.

Helpful Hints and Precautions:

As in Ardha Shalabasana, avoid bending knees, stiffening calves, and pointing toes. Keep your chin and shoulders in contact with the ground throughout the posture. The most advanced stage of this posture requires utmost strength and flexibility in lumbar spinal muscles. Before raising legs, be sure that the whole weight of the body rests on the chest and arms.

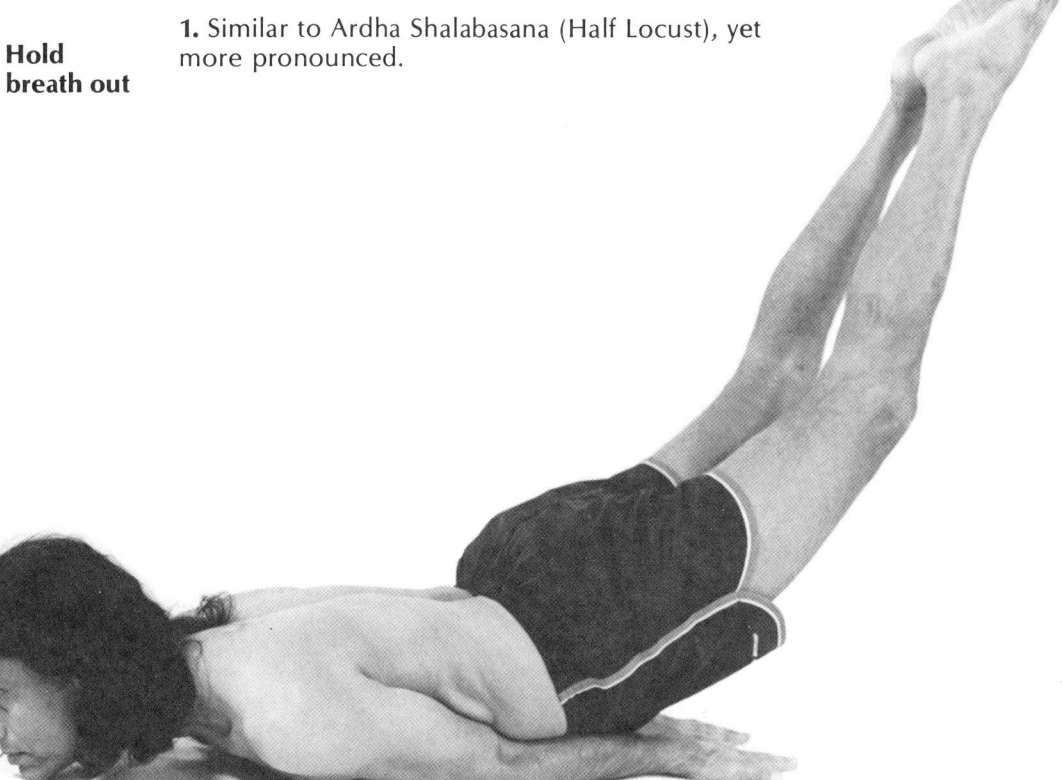

PASCHIMOTTANASANA—POSTERIOR STRETCH

Technique:

1. Sit on the floor with your legs outstretched in front of you. Place your palms on the floor beside the hips.

2. Raise your arms sideways and upwards while stretching and lifting your chest and abdomen from the waist. Relax your shoulders.

Inhale

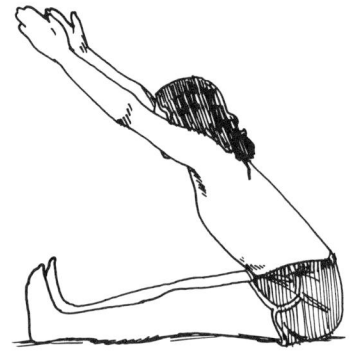

3. Begin to stretch forward by rotating from the hinge of your hip joints, lengthening your spine without bending at the waist. Extend your arms from the shoulders.

Exhale

4. Stretch forward only so far as is comfortable without lifting your knees or rounding your back. Hold.

Breathe

5. Grasp onto either ankles or toes or clasp hands around the soles of your feet (wherever you can reach), while maintaining a straight spine and keeping your knees on the floor. Hold.

Breathe deeply

6. Bend the elbows, using them as levers to help gravity pull your torso forward as you lengthen the muscles at the back of your thighs.

Exhale forward

7. Maintain the position for sixty seconds.

Breathe deeply

8. Release your hands, and slowly begin to raise your torso and arms upward, keeping your spine straight.

Inhale slowly

9. Lower your arms sideways to the floor and relax.

Exhale slowly

Benefits of Paschimottanasana:

1. Keeps abdominal organs free from sluggishness, through compression.

2. Tones kidneys by stretching the back.

3. Stretches, tones, and lengthens entire spinal column.

4. Due to the extra stretch given to the pelvic region, brings more oxygenated blood to the sexual organs, thereby helping these organs to absorb nutrition from the blood, which increases vitality and ultimately leads to greater sexual control.

5. Provides a powerful stretch for the entire back of the body from the heels to the back of the neck.

6. Deeply tranquilizes the whole system, calming mind and emotions.

Helpful Hints and Precautions:

When the posture is done properly, no weight should be felt on your back. Concentrate on stretching from the pelvic region of your back rather than from your upper back and shoulders.

If you suffer from back injury or severe constipation, practice Paschimottanasana (Posterior Stretch) carefully, gradually increasing the length of your holding time.

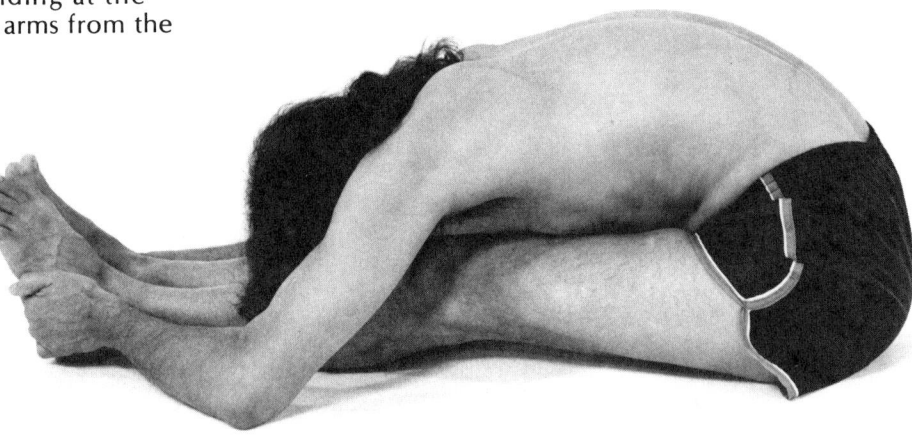

PURVOTTANASANA—INCLINED PLANE

Technique:

1. Sit on floor, legs together and extended in front of you, palms flat on the floor behind you, fingers pointing away from your body.

2. Lean back slightly on your hands.

3. Press down on your palms and raise your hips as high as you can. Bring your feet down flat on the floor. Contract your buttocks and flatten the lower back by pressing the pubic bone upward.

Inhale up

4. Drop your head back.

Exhale

5. Hold the posture, being sure to keep your legs straight and your toes pointed downward. Hold for at least the length of several deep inhalations and exhalations.

Breathe normally

Benefits of Purvottanasana:

1. Provides stretch and lengthening to the entire front of the body.

2. Helps firm abdomen, hip and thighs.

3. Strengthens wrists.

Helpful Hints and Precautions:

When you drop your head back it stretches the whole front of your body from head to heels. Once you can raise your hips high enough, your spine and back will share in body support. You can also point your fingers toward your body which will provide a different stretch in the shoulders. The higher you push your hips, the more you stretch and strengthen the legs, shoulders and arms.

This posture is a counterpose to Paschimottanasana (Posterior Stretch).

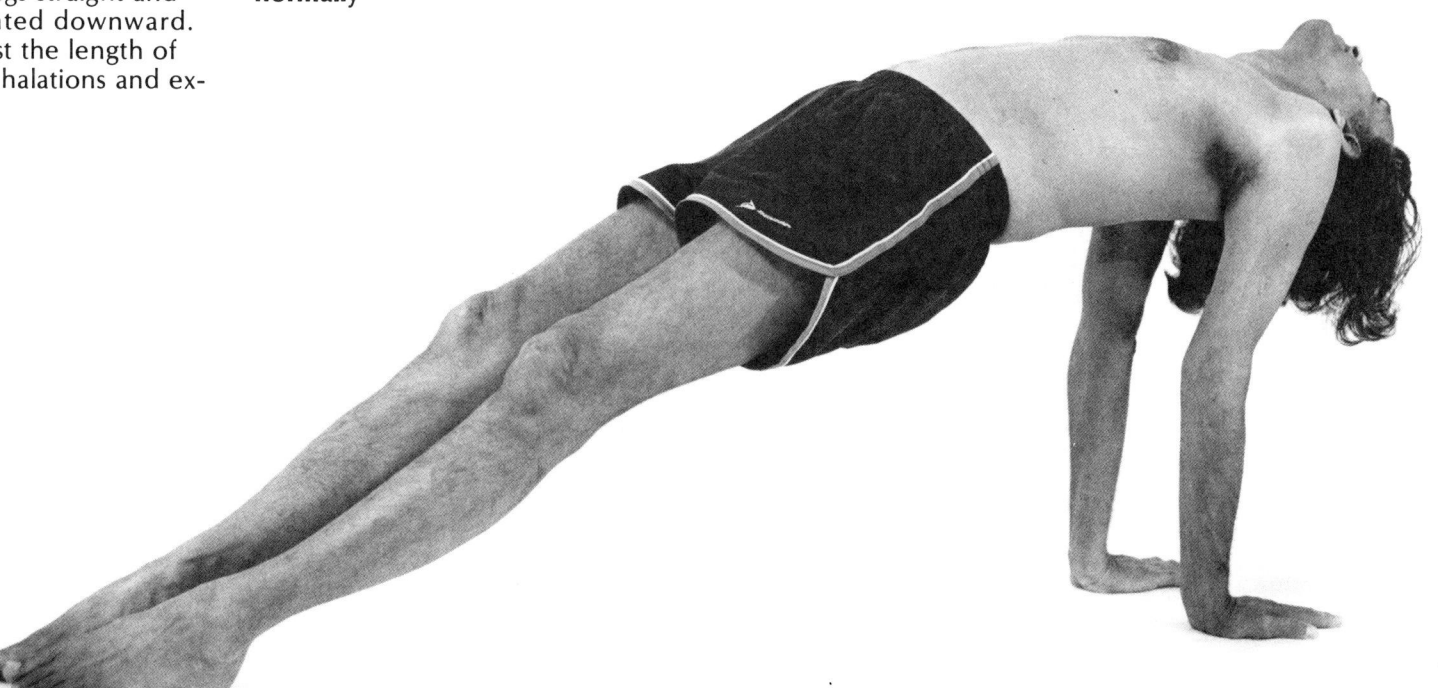

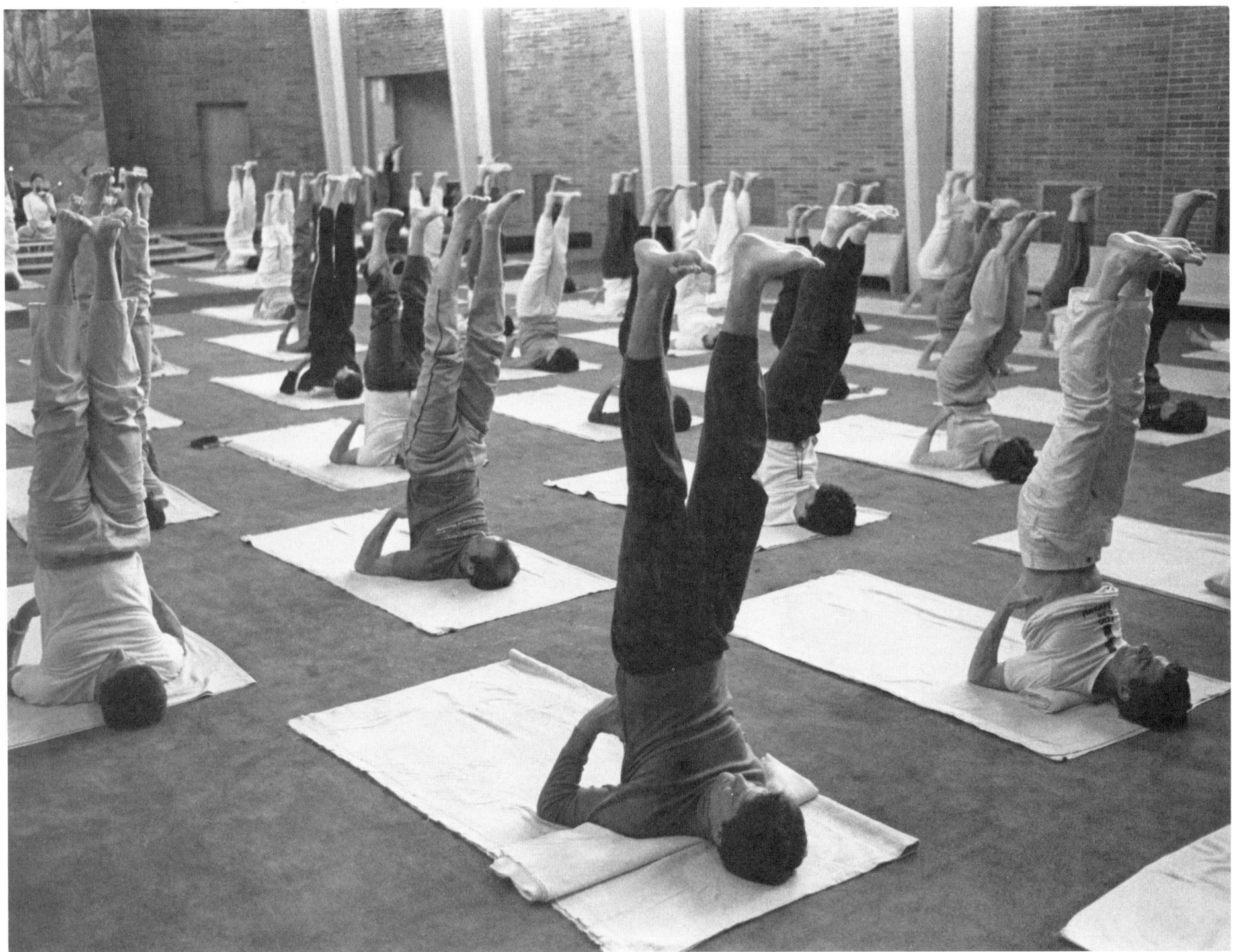

SARVANGASANA—SHOULDERSTAND

Technique:

1. Lie flat on your back with your legs outstretched. Align your body, as in Tadasana (Mountain) with your feet flexed, kneecaps lifted, and your tail-bone tucked under. Place your arms by your sides, palms facing the floor. **Breathe deeply**

2. Lift your outstretched legs towards the ceiling. **Exhale**

3. Raise your hips from the floor, lifting your torso so that it is perpendicular to the floor. Support your back by placing your hands on either side of the middle of your back. **Inhale**

4. Hold. **Breathe deeply**

5. Slowly walk your hands toward your shoulder blades to fully straighten and extend your spine, thereby lifting your chest toward your chin. Shift from side to side and bring the elbows as close together behind you as possible. Your weight is thus supported fully by your shoulders and upper arms with the back of your head and neck free.

6. Alternately flex and point your feet as you hold Sarvangasana, stretching and working both sides of your legs. **Ujjayi breath**

7. Release the posture by lowering your knees toward your forehead, legs straight, placing your arms palms down on the floor behind you, and slowly roll your spine down, vertebra by vertebra, until your entire spine is on the floor. **Breathe normally**

8. Slowly straighten and lower your legs to the floor. **Breathe normally**

9. Relax. **Breathe normally**

Benefits of Sarvangasana:

1. Helps correct weight problems due to metabolic imbalances by normalizing the function of the thyroid and parathyroid glands situated in the throat, which due to the firm chin-lock receive an increased blood supply when posture is released.

2. Improves venous circulation, relieving pressure on the blood vessels and making them resilient. Prevents and can relieve varicose veins and hemorrhoids.

3. Because of the inverted posture, stimulates the abdominal organs, freeing the movement of the bowels, and allows blood from the legs and trunk to flow to the heart without gravitational strain.

4. Greatly relieves ailments of the neck and chest by increasing the circulation in those areas.

5. Corrects displacement of vital internal glands and organs, especially the female organs. Benefits those suffering from female disorders.

6. Tones the gonads, maintaining the vitality of the entire body. Restores dissipated energy, bringing new youth to the entire system.

7. Nourishes facial skin, scalp, and hair roots, improving general complexion.

Helpful Hints and Precautions:

The Shoulderstand is a precious gift given to humanity by the ancient yogis. Its Sanskrit name means "The exercise that benefits the entire body." It produces many of the rejuvenating effects of the more difficult inverted postures, such as the Headstand.

Individuals suffering from high or low blood pressure, chronic thyroid disorders, chronic nasal catarrah, glaucoma, detached retina, or weak eye capillaries should consult a physician before attempting the Shoulderstand.

Individuals with known cervical and shoulder strain should proceed with extreme caution, consulting a physician.

HALASANA—PLOW

Technique:

1. Go into Sarvangasana (Shoulder-stand) with a firm chin-lock.

2. Bend from your hips, lowering your legs to stretch over your head. Allow your flexed feet to reach as close to the floor as possible without bending the spine. Bend only from your hips.   **Exhale**

3. Place your hands in the middle of your back, applying pressure to keep your torso perpendicular to the floor.

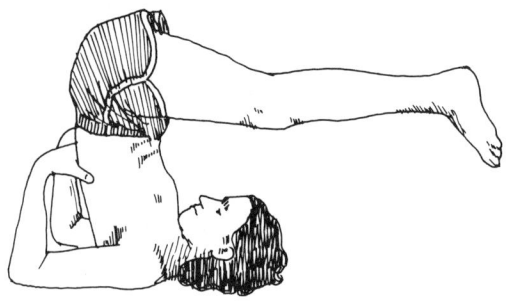

4. Keep your legs straight by flexing your feet.

5. Stretch your arms on the floor in the opposite direction of your legs, interlocking the fingers behind your back.

6. Hold in this position.   **Breathe deeply**

7. Release your hands.   **Inhale**

8. Replace your hands on your back and slowly raise the body back into Sarvangasana.   **Slow exhalation**

9. Gradually release back onto the floor.   **Continue to exhale**

10. Relax for several breaths.   **Normal breath**

Benefits of Halasana:

1. Stretches the entire back of the body from the nape of the neck to the heels. Aligns the vertebrae and brings a fresh supply of blood to the nerve centers along the spine.

2. Relieves backaches due to relaxation of the spine and back muscles.

3. Relieves cramping in hands and fingers through interlocking and stretching of palms and fingers.

4. Brings flexibility and strength to the arms, neck, and shoulders, thereby releasing tension in these areas.

5. Enhances body symmetry and strengthens the back muscles.

6. Brings greater strength and mobility to the back, and makes Paschimottanasana (Posterior Stretch) easier to perform.

7. Massages and stimulates abdominal organs through contraction.

8. Relieves gas in stomach.

9. Trims accumulation of fat from the abdomen and hips. Tones and firms the legs.

10. Helps regulate the functions of thyroid, calming nerves and blessing the entire system with youthfulness.

11. Rejuvenates and cleanses the gonads, pancreas, liver, spleen, kidneys, and supra-renal glands.

12. Relieves exhaustion, fatigue, and stiffness of the back and shoulders. Aids treatment of menstrual disorders.

13. Increases circulation to the brain, stimulating brain activity; clears the mind.

Helpful Hints and Precautions:

If Halasana is initially difficult for you, try this simple preparation: lie on the floor with the top of your head about 18" from a wall; then simply walk feet down the wall to the floor. Be careful not to overstrain by overly vigorous or jerky movements. Do not attempt to force your toes to the floor; it is more important to keep your spine extended and straight, bending only from your hips.

Persons with high blood pressure should not do the Plow.

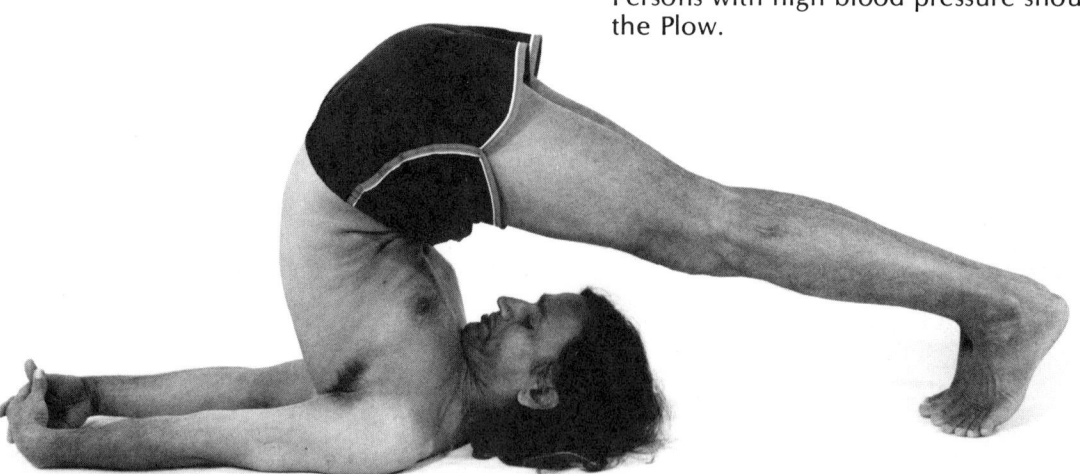

MATSYASANA—FISH & SUPTA VAJRASANA—FISH SUPINE

Technique:

1. Lie on your back with legs out-stretched, feet together. Breathe comfortably. For an advanced classical variation place your legs in Lotus position (Padmasana).

2. Place your elbows on the floor close to your sides. Pushing down on your elbows, lift your chest and rest on the crown of your head, creating an arch in your back.

3. Gradually lift your lower, middle and upper back, pressing your hips toward the ceiling, lifting your sternum until your weight is supported by your head and feet.

Exhale

4. Continue to hold.

Breathe deeply

5. If you can comfortably release the elbow support, place your hands in prayer position over your chest during the holding phase.

6. To return, press elbows into the floor, lower your head and then your back to rest on the floor.

Exhale

Advanced Variation:
Supta Vajrasana—Fish Supine

1. From Sarvangasana (Shoulderstand), with your hands firmly supporting your back, arch backwards. Bend and lower one leg at a time, placing your feet on the floor behind you—moving into Setu Bandhasana (Bridge) with your weight supported by your shoulders and feet.

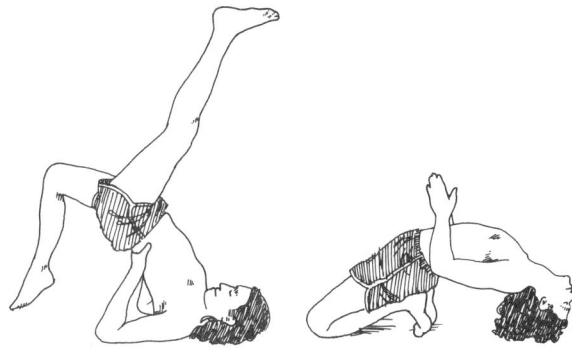

2. Fold your lowered legs under you and rest your buttocks on your heels. (For even more stretch, keep your toes curled under.) At the same time, using your forearms for support, arch your upper back and rest the crown of your head on the floor.

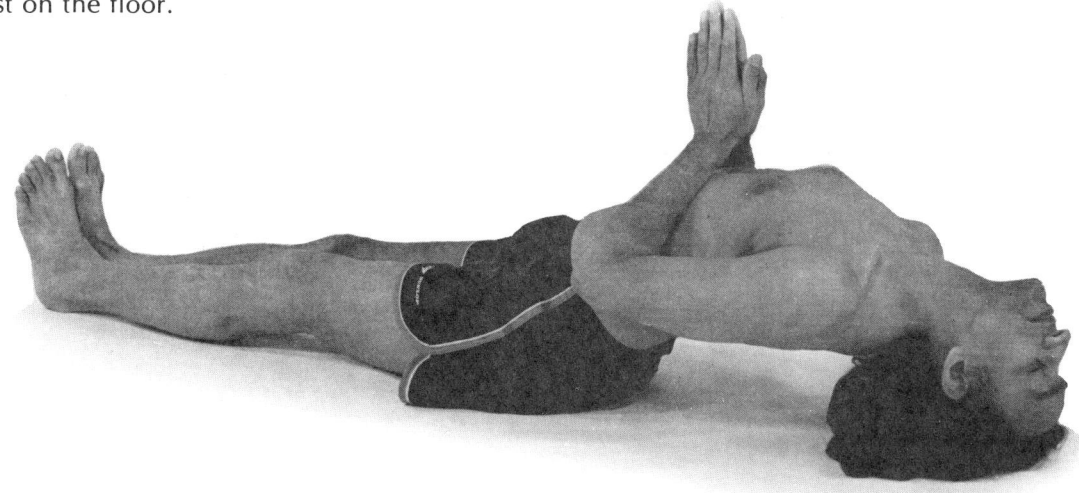

3. If you can comfortably release the elbow support, place your hands in prayer position over your chest as you hold the posture.

4. To return, bring elbows back to the floor, lower your head, straighten your legs, and relax with your back on the floor.

Benefits of Matsyasana:

1. Counterbalances the action of Sarvangasana (Shoulderstand) by arching the nape of the neck and giving it freedom. Brings about thoracic and clavicular breathing because the upper lobes of the lungs and the region under the collarbone receive more air.

2. Gives excellent abdominal stretch, decongesting that area.

3. Stimulates the pancreas, aids in relief of hypoglycemic symptoms, and prevents diabetes.

4. Effectively loosens rounded, stiffened areas of the back, particularly the shoulder blade region.

5. Brings to the muscles of the spine an increased supply of blood which spreads to the spinal cord, increasing elasticity and soothing the sympathetic nervous system.

6. Stimulates pelvic organs, particularly genitals and ovaries.

7. Brings tone to the adrenals, normalizing adrenalin production.

8. If done in Padmasana (Lotus), diverts circulation in the legs to the base of the abdomen, greatly benefiting the gonads.

Helpful Hints and Precautions:

If doing Matsyasana in its classical form, during Padmasana (Lotus), be sure to switch leg positions so each leg has a chance to be on top for equal holding duration. Only perform in Padmasana if you can do so with ease.

SETU BANDHASANA — BRIDGE

Technique:

1. Lie on your back with your knees bent, your feet placed hip-width apart and close to your buttocks, grounded as in Tadasana (Mountain), and if possible grasp your ankles with your hands.

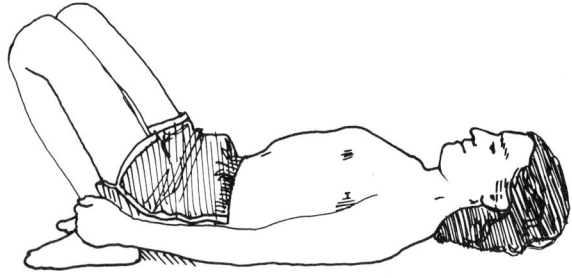

2. To engage your body, press your lower back into the floor by contracting the buttocks and tucking your tailbone under.

3. Gradually lift your lower, middle, and upper back, pressing your hips toward the ceiling. Lift your sternum until your weight is supported by your shoulders and feet.

4. Hold.

5. Release the posture by slowly lowering your spine one vertebra at a time back onto the floor.

6. Relax and breathe normally.

Benefits of Setu Bandhasana:

1. Increases flexibility in your spine and shoulders.

2. Strengthens the muscles of your abdomen and thighs during the holding.

3. Relieves pressure on the neck sometimes felt during Sarvangasana (Shoulderstand) and Halasana (Plow).

Helpful Hints and Precautions:

Setu Bandhasana may also be done by placing your hands on either side of your back, as in Sarvangasana (Shoulderstand) in order to help support the spine in the arch. To protect your thumbs, keep your hands in the same position as in Sarvangasana (Shoulderstand) with your thumbs to the outside. For an advanced sequence, you may do Sarvangasana (Shoulderstand), Halasana (Plow), Setu Bandhasana (Bridge), and Supta Vajrasana (Fish Supine) as one continuous series.

Kapalabhati

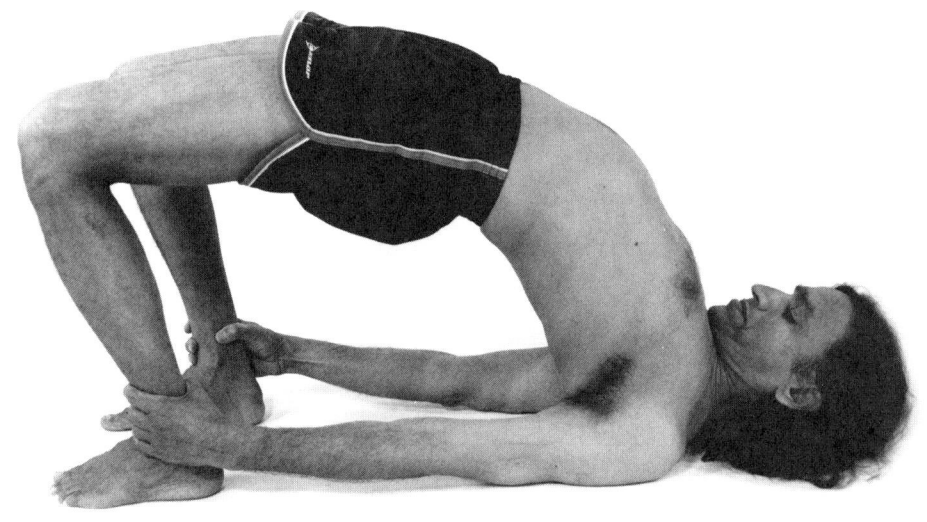

CHAKRASANA—WHEEL

Technique:

1. Lie on your back with your knees bent, feet close to your buttocks and lined up with your hips. Place your hands beneath your shoulders, fingers pointing toward your feet, and elbows toward the ceiling. Tuck your tailbone under.

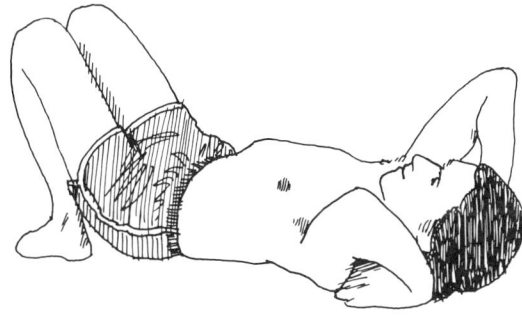

2. Press down on your hands, lift your hips to arch your back and place the top of your head on the floor.

Inhale

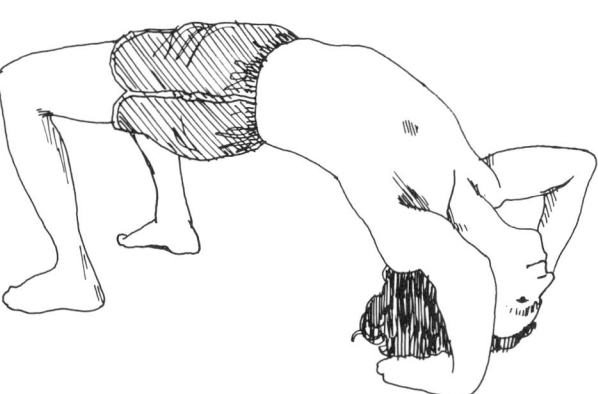

3. Continue lifting your hips as you straighten your arms, and lift your head from the floor. Straighten your legs. Your weight is thus supported by your feet and hands.

4. Hold the position.

5. Release by bending both your knees and arms and lowering your head back to the floor and slowly uncurling your spine to return to the floor.

6. Relax.

Exhale

Kapalabhati 15 x

Exhale

Breathe normally

Benefits of Chakrasana:

1. As an intense back-bending posture, energizes the whole body and leaves a feeling of lightness.

2. Tones the spine and helps to keep the whole body flexible.

3. Strengthens the arms, legs, and abdomen.

Helpful Hints and Precautions:

If this position is too difficult, practice Setu Bandhasana (Bridge) until you develop more strength in your arms and legs.

In Step 3, to help experience a greater lift and stretch across your abdomen, come onto your toes, and then lower your heels, resting your weight on your soles and hands.

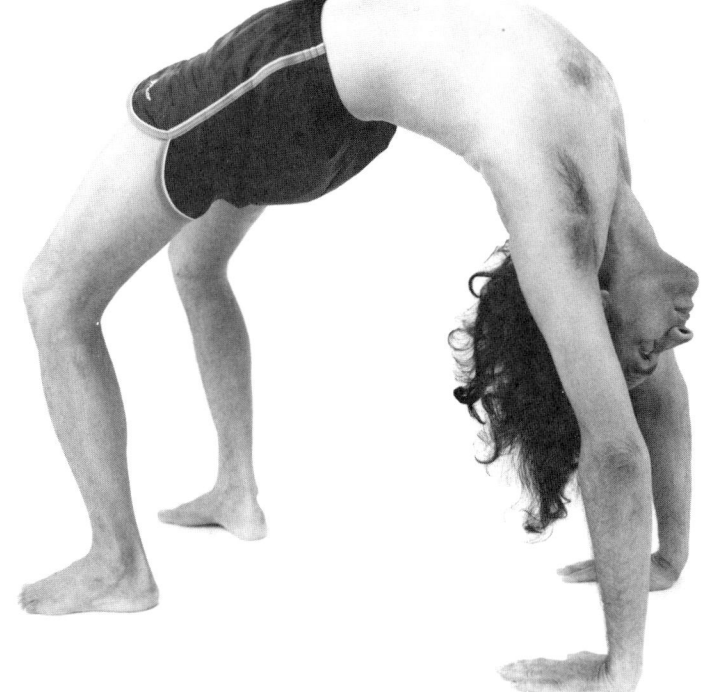

MATSYENDRASANA—SPINAL TWIST

Technique:

1. Sit in a kneeling position with your knees together.

2. Shift your hips so that you sit to the left of your feet.

3. Lift your right leg over your left, placing your right foot against the outside of the left knee.

4. Bring your right heel in close to your buttocks, keeping your spine erect. Establish evenness in your seat between both sides of your buttocks.

5. Stretch your arms out sideways, perpendicular to your torso. Begin to twist to the right.   **Exhale**

6. Bring the left arm down to the outside of the right knee, grasping the right foot. Place the right hand on the floor behind your hips or around your waist. (Variation: Place the left arm through the window of your right bent leg and bring your right hand around your waist, clasping your left hand.)   **Inhale**

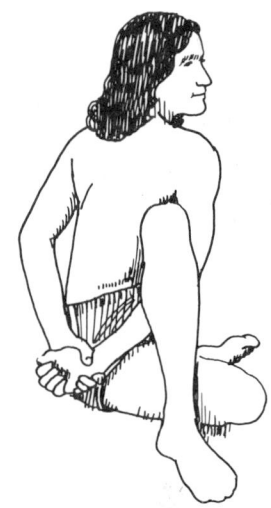

7. Continue twisting the body as far as possible. Turn your navel to the right, and turn your sternum, your shoulders, neck, head, and eyes to look over your right shoulder. Keep your chin parallel to your shoulders, and your shoulders in line with your upper knee.   **Exhale**

8. Hold for 60 seconds.   **Breathe normally**

9. Reverse steps, first returning your head forward, then releasing arms and hands.   **Inhale**

10. Repeat entire posture in the opposite direction.

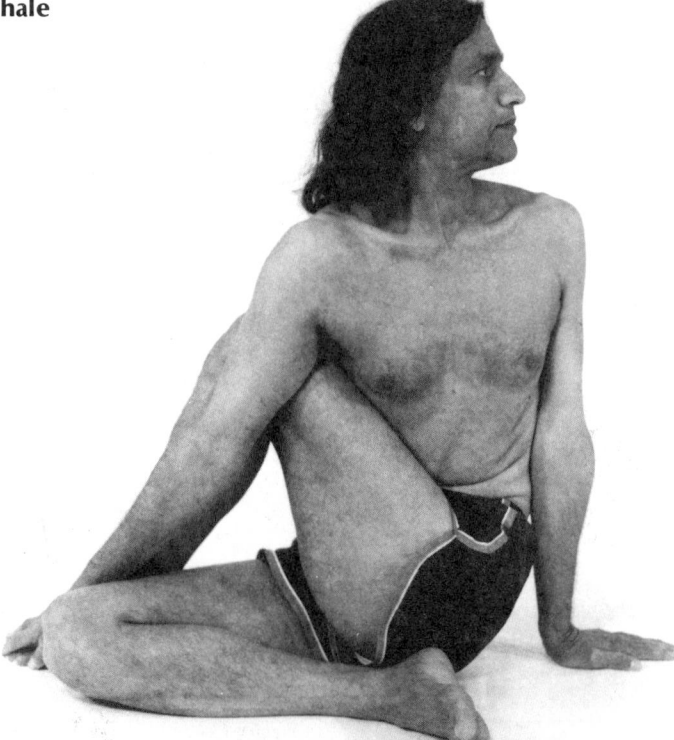

Benefits of Matsyendrasana:

1. Rotates and fully extends the spine (unlike most postures, which only bend it backward or forward).

2. Through the twist to the spine, tones and strengthens the spinal nerves, and creates a sense of well-being.

3. Activates organs in lower abdomen due to the squeeze given by the thigh pressing into that area.

4. Aids elimination by pressure applied first to the right side and then to the left side, progressing in the direction of peristalsis.

5. Affects the ascending colon and activates the liver and gall bladder (located on the right side of the body below the rib cage) and the right kidney through the pressure of the bent right leg.

6. Affects the descending colon and activates the stomach, spleen and the left kidney through the pressure of the bent left leg.

7. Removes calcium deposits in the shoulders, freeing shoulder movement. Overcomes stiffness of the neck.

8. Hydrates the intervertebral spinal discs and provides fresh blood and oxygen to entire skeletal muscular system along the spine.

9. Corrects curvature of spine (scoliosis) created by imbalanced pull of postural muscles on spine.

10. Good antidote for those who either sit or stand for a long time.

Helpful Hints and Precautions:

Keep your back extended and straight while twisting to prevent any injury to the spine.

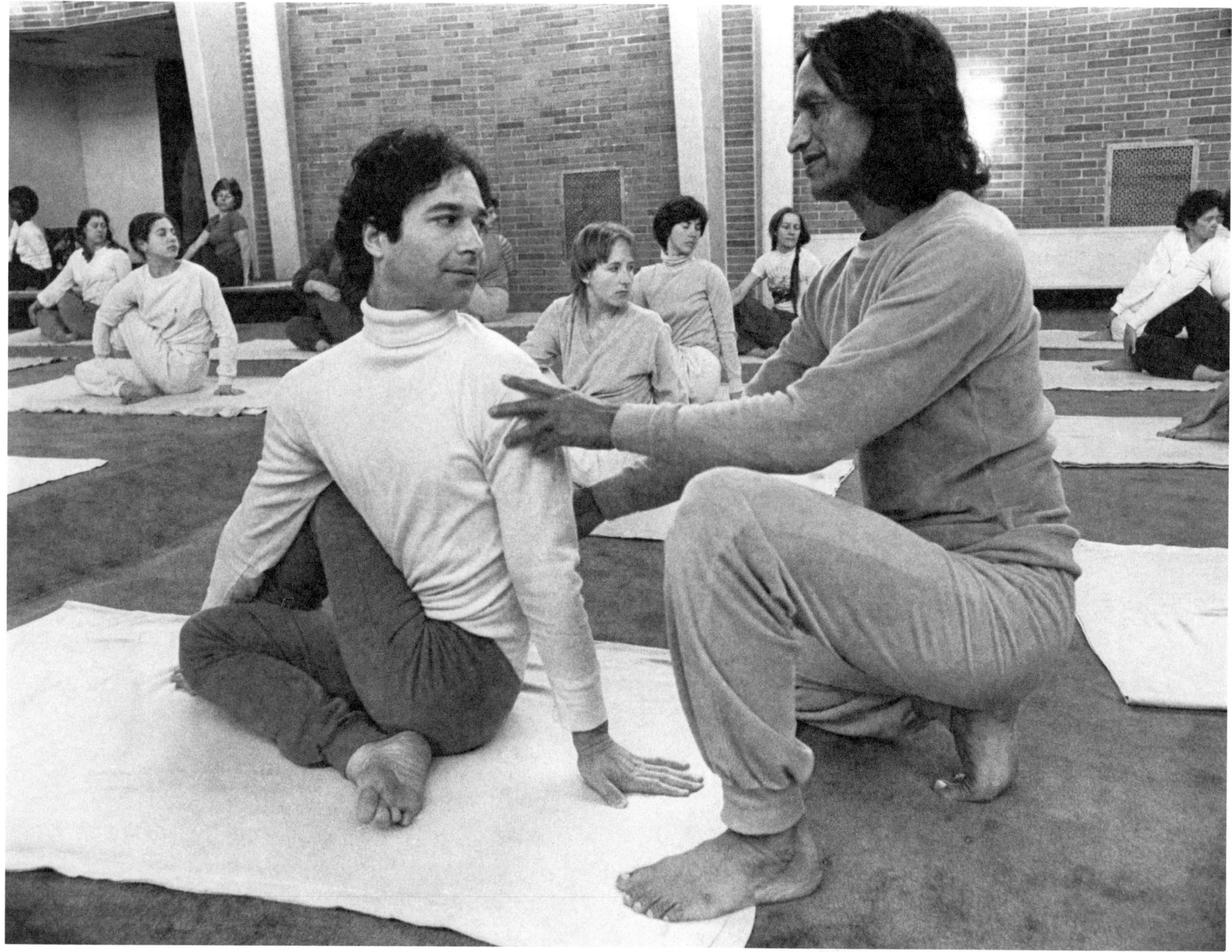

VIRASANA—HERO

Technique:

1. Kneeling, cross your legs so that the right knee is on top of the left knee. Place hands on feet.

2. Move your feet away from your hips until you feel a hip stretch. You will increase the stretch to your hips by moving your feet further away from your hips.   **Inhale deeply**

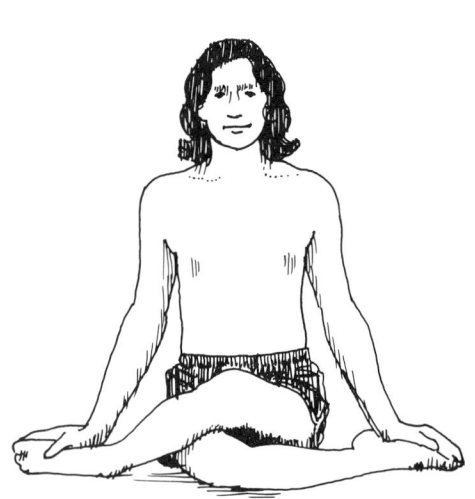

3. Place the palms of your hands on the soles of your feet and bend your upper body forward.   **Exhale**

4. Hold.   **Breathe normally**

5. Return to sitting.   **Exhale**

6. Repeat, starting with the left knee on top of the right knee.

Benefits of Virasana:

1. Opens the hip area, allowing your legs to move more freely at the hip joint.

2. By placing the right knee on top, through pressure in the direction of peristalsis, affects the ascending colon, and activates the liver and gall bladder (located on the right side of the body below the rib cage) and the right kidney.

3. By placing the left knee on top, affects the descending colon, the spleen (located on the left side below the rib cage) and the left kidney.

4. Aids the body in removal of calcium deposits from the shoulders, freeing shoulder movement. Overcomes stiffness of the neck.

Helpful Hints and Precautions:

For greatest benefit, do this posture along with Matsyendrasana, the Spinal Twist.

Bend your upper body forward only if you can sit comfortably with your legs in this knee-over-knee position.

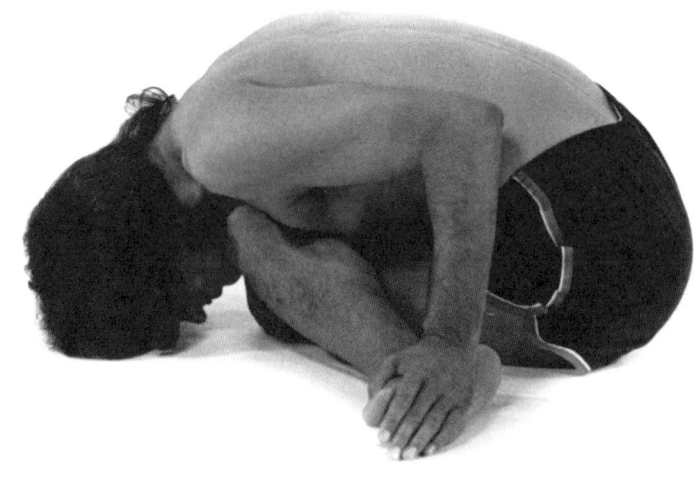

SHIRSHASANA—HEADSTAND

Technique:

1. Kneel on the floor. Lean forward, placing your elbows on the floor (the distance between your elbows should be the same as the distance from your elbow to your hand). Clasp your hands to make a cup with your fingers and to form a tripod between your hands and elbows.

2. Rest the top of your head, not your forehead, on the floor, with the cup of your hands around the back of your head.

3. Curl your toes under, raise your hips and straighten your legs, supporting your weight with your elbows and wrists. Keep your shoulders up and back.

4. Slowly walk your feet toward your body and lift high in the hips (this brings your hips into the proper position to balance the Headstand).

5. When your hips are in the proper position for balance, your knees will naturally tend to bend. Gently lift one knee in toward the chest and then the other. Do not kick up into the Headstand.

6. Raise your thighs by using the strength of your arms and hand grip so that your feet are directly above your hips.

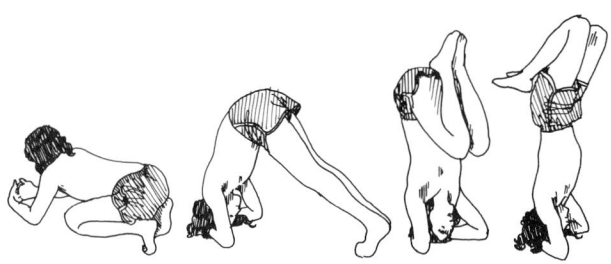

7. Slowly straighten your legs toward the ceiling. Be sure not to arch your back as you raise into Shirshasana. Keep your tailbone tucked under. As you hold the position, continue to lift up out of the shoulders and from the soles of your relaxed feet.

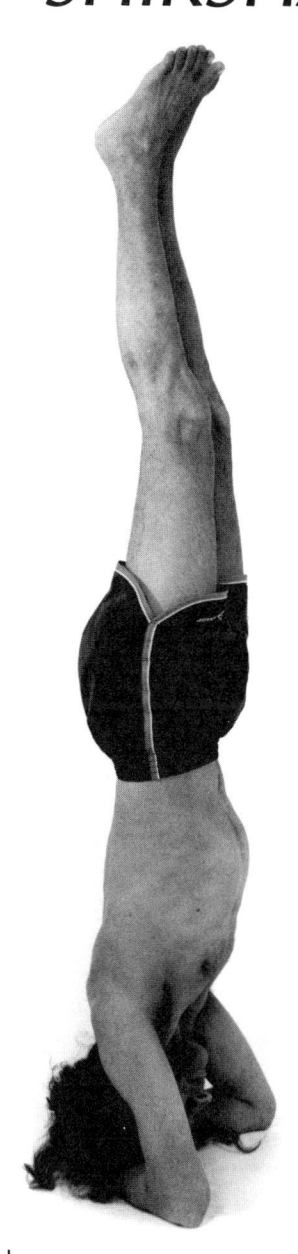

8. To come down, reverse your upward movement.

9. Rest in Garbhasana (the Child Pose) for a few moments with your forehead resting on your fists.

Benefits of Shirshasana:

1. Energizes the whole body.

2. Cleanses the brain by flushing the capillaries and blood vessels, relieving headaches, migraines, and nervous fatigue, and improving memory, concentration, and intellectual capacity.

3. Helps normalize the functions of the pituitary and pineal glands, which control the endocrine system.

4. Improves eyesight and hearing.

5. Regenerates and smooths the skin and scalp.

6. Helps relieve colds, infections of the tonsils and adrenal glands, constipation, poor circulation, female disorders, and the overall lack of self-confidence or vitality.

7. Improves posture.

Helpful Hints and Precautions:

The Headstand is known as the "king of the asanas". It is unrivaled for the extent of its physical, mental, and emotional benefits. With consistent practice, students of any age can master this posture. It is not necessary, however, to perform the Headstand in order to derive the full benefits of yoga. Proceed at your own speed. By being patient with yourself, you will achieve success.

Practice the Headstand on a firm, but thick carpet or mat. Do not use a soft pillow or cushion, as this will make balancing difficult. You may prefer to use a wall to support your back and legs before attempting the posture in the middle of the room.

The Headstand should not be done by anyone with a detached retina, organically defective pineal or pituitary gland, eye disease, or infected ears. In case of extremely high or low blood pressure, consult a physician first. Remember to remove rings and contact lenses.

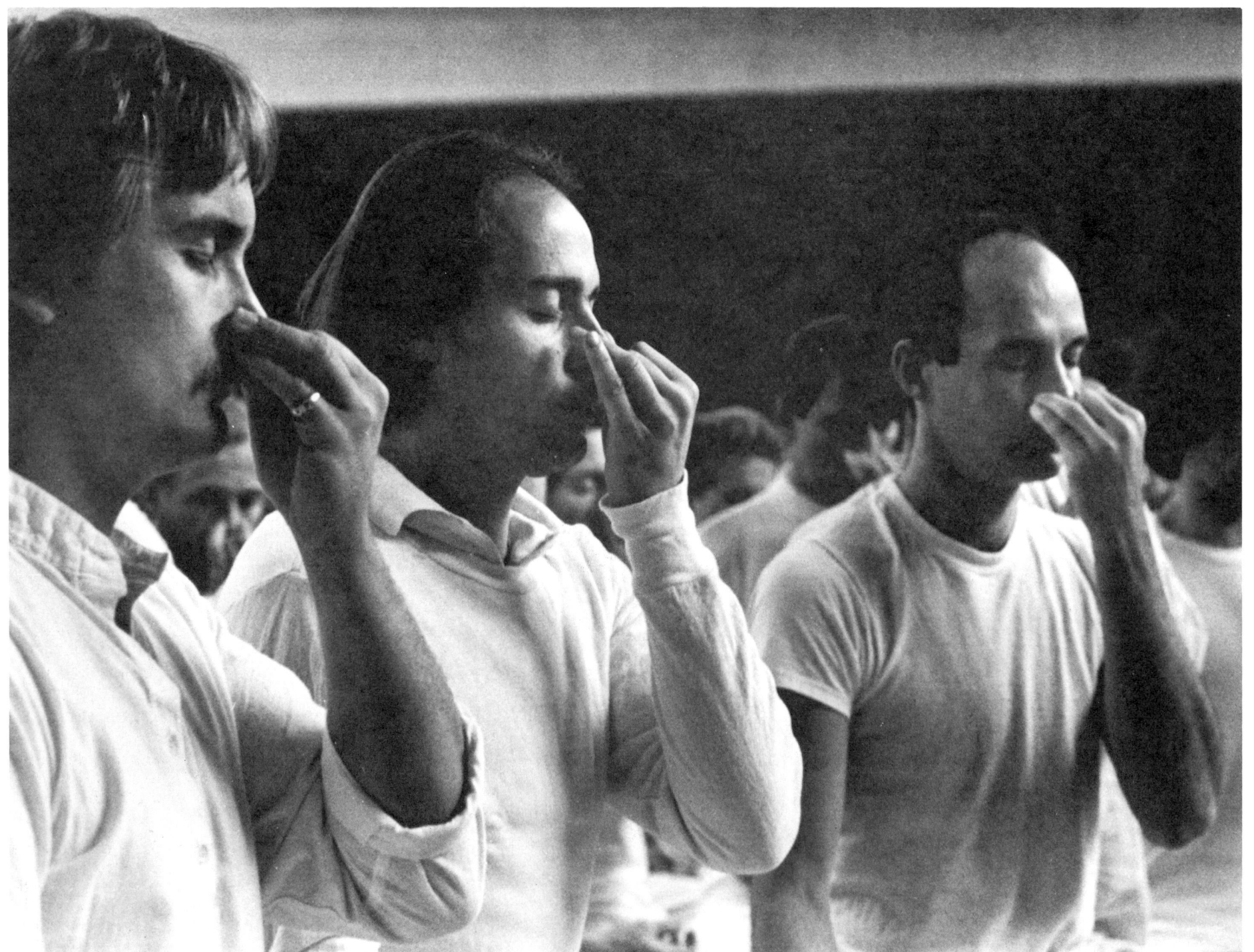

Pranayama and Other Techniques

Here we present step-by-step directions for each technique that accompanies the postures above. It is suggested that you carefully read the instructions for a given exercise before you perform it. In the practice of pranayama, the following points are helpful to remember:

1. I recommend daily aerobic exercise as a simple, natural way to stimulate deep breathing and to prepare your body for pranayama.

2. Diet has a profound effect on pranayama. Notice which foods produce excessive mucus in your system, and consider reducing or eliminating those foods from your diet, for better breath control and enhanced benefits. Dairy products are a common cause of excessive mucus for some people.

3. Breathe in and out in a smooth, uniform flow. Avoid irregular and jerky movements.

4. When you hold your breath, do so comfortably, without straining; strained holding prevents control during exhalation.

5. Avoid tensing unrelated muscles. If tension persists, reread the directions to make sure that you are following them properly.

6. Once you have mastered the postures, you may keep your attention on the breath and observe its effects on various parts of your body. This trains the mind to remain concentrated, alert, and steady. Control and concentration of the mind are necessary for higher stages of Kripalu Yoga.

COMPLETE YOGIC BREATH

Technique:

1. Lie comfortably in Shavasana (Corpse Pose): flat on your back with your legs spread about a foot apart, arms by your sides, palms upwards. Relax your body completely. Exhale fully.

2. Inhale deeply through your nose. Allow your relaxed stomach to expand like an inflated balloon.

3. Exhale through your nose, and contract your stomach muscles until the diaphragm expands and presses upward into the thoracic cavity under the ribs.

4. Continue breathing until you have established a natural rhythm. Notice your abdomen rise and fall.

5. Repeat this abdominal breathing five to ten times.

6. After one week of practice, continue to breathe abdominally, but add the following: after filling your lower lungs, concentrate on filling first your middle lungs, and then your upper lungs. As you exhale, first deflate your upper lungs, then your middle lungs, and then deflate the abdomen. Make your breath steady and rhythmic, like a wave rising and flowing in, and then flowing out again. This is the Complete Yogic Breath.

Benefits of Complete Yogic Breath:

1. Relaxes the entire body and nervous system, particularly the abdominal region where we hold so many tensions and anxieties.

2. Relaxes the heart, reducing blood pressure.

3. Massages the abdomen, toning the organs, stimulating digestion, regulating intestinal activity and elimination.

4. Provides relief for respiratory problems.

5. Regular practice increases the amount of air taken in with each inhalation, using more of the lungs, resulting in more oxygen intake from each breath, and hence slower respiration. This bestows calmness to the body and increased clarity to the mind.

6. Helps calm emotions.

Helpful Hints and Precautions:

The objective of this exercise is to establish a new breath pattern of deep, full, even breaths. Many people have acquired the habit of very shallow breathing which uses only part of their lungs, resulting in less oxygen than desirable.

Begin by lying on the floor. Once the technique is mastered, practice in an erect sitting position. The technique can also be used standing or walking. It is desirable that this breath pattern gradually become habitual throughout the day.

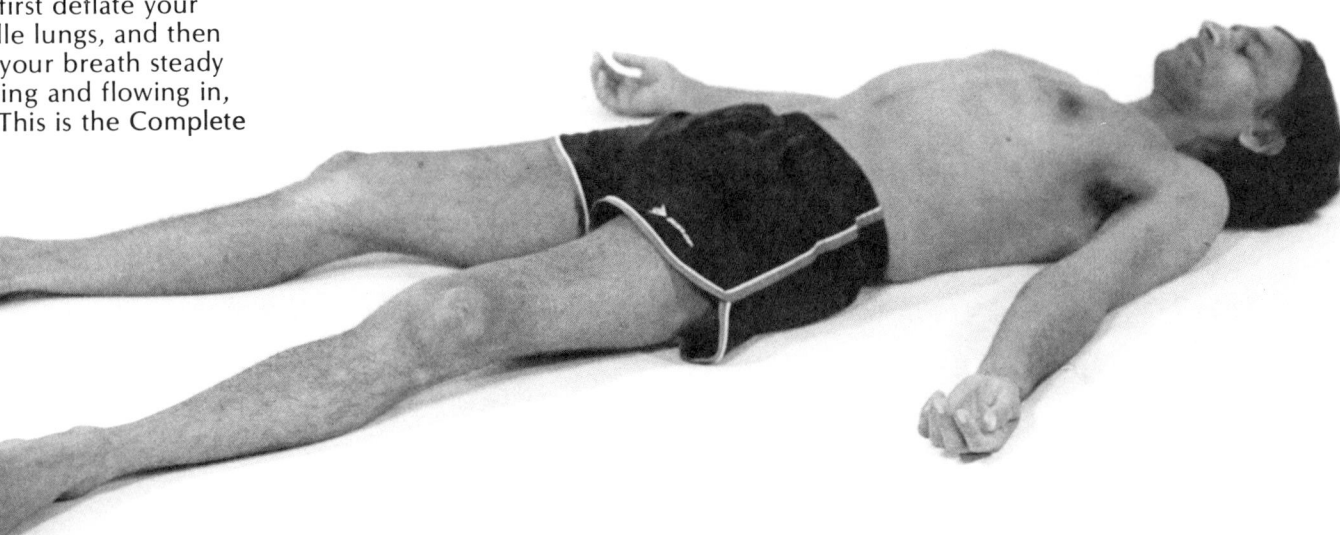

UJJAYI—SOUNDING BREATH

Technique:

1. Lie comfortably in Shavasana (Corpse Pose): flat on your back, legs spread slightly apart, arms at your sides with palms up.

2. Inhale through your nose, drawing your breath in slowly. Contract the back of your throat slightly as if making an "ahhh" sound, but with the mouth closed. This will create a slight hissing sound at constriction at the back of the throat as the air passes over the windpipe. Contracting the back of your throat also lets you regulate the flow of your breath, thereby allowing you to prolong the inhalation and exhalation.

3. As you continue with the slow inhalation, let your abdomen relax and expand in the Complete Yogic Breath (see above).

4. Continue to contract the back of the throat slightly as if making an "eeee" sound, with the mouth closed, while you exhale. Exhale as you slowly pull the abdomen in and up to fully empty your lungs. Control the flow of your breath: let it be long and slow.

5. Continue to inhale and exhale in this way.

KAPALABHATI

In Kapalabhati, the exhalation is forced, the inhalation spontaneous. There is a split second of retention after each exhalation.

Technique:

1. Exhale vigorously through the nose; at the same time pull in your abdomen; then allow the inhalation to happen passively by relaxing your abdomen. This is one round.

2. Repeat in a steady rhythmic series of exhalations according to your capacity. Emphasize the exhalation each time.

3. Variation: Instead of using both nostrils you may alternate nostrils, closing off right nostril then left nostril with alternate exhalations.

Benefits of Kapalabhati:

1. Cleanses and purifies the entire respiratory system by forcing air from the extremities of the lungs.

2. By increasing the amount of oxygen in the system, clears the mind and improves concentration.

Helpful Hints and Precautions:

Kapalabhati can be practiced at the end of each round of Agnisara Dhauti (Abdominal Pumps) to quickly regain natural breathing. This practice is forceful and is strenuous for those with weak lungs and weak constitutions. It is contraindicated for those with ear infections or glaucoma, and for those with high blood pressure. If nose begins to bleed, or ears ache or throb, discontinue for a while.

ANULOM VILOMA—ALTERNATE NOSTRIL BREATH

Basically, in this breathing technique you inhale through one nostril, retain the breath, then exhale through the other nostril in a 1:4:2 ratio. As an example we will use the count 2:8:4.

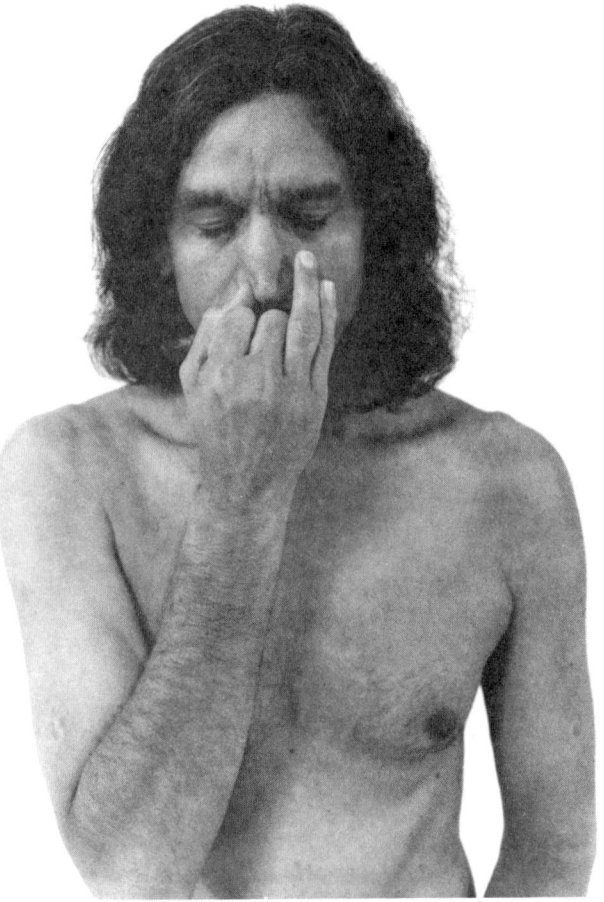

Technique:

1. Sit comfortably.

2. Place your right hand in the Vishnu mudra (tuck index and middle fingers into palm). Bring your hand close to your nostrils. Use the thumb to close off the right nostril and the third and fourth fingers to close off the left nostril.

3. Close the right nostril with your thumb and breathe in through the left nostril to the count of two.

4. Hold the breath, closing both nostrils to the count of eight.

5. Keep the left nostril closed with your third and fourth fingers. Breathe out through the right nostril to the count of four.

6. Keep the left nostril closed and breathe in through the right nostril to the count of two.

7. Hold the breath, closing both nostrils to the count of eight.

8. Keep the right nostril closed with your thumb and breathe out through the left nostril to the count of four.

The above procedure constitutes one round of Anulom Viloma.

9. You can increase the duration of inhalation, holding, and exhalation as comfort allows, keeping the same ratio (i.e. 3:12:6, 4:16:8, 5:20:10). For counting, you can use guru mantra.

Benefits of Anulom Viloma:

1. Anulom Viloma plays a powerful role in awakening prana. During the retention of breath in Anulom Viloma you can simultaneously apply the Chin Lock, Jalandhara Bandha, as given on the following page.

2. Restores a balanced flow of prana to the body. (A healthy person breathes predominately through the left nostril for one hour fifty minutes and then through the right. Anulom Viloma will restore this natural breathing rhythm, which is disturbed in many people.)

3. Has a calming, stilling, balancing effect on the mind, helping one to more readily enter meditation.

JALANDHARA BANDHA—CHIN LOCK

Technique:

1. Sit with the spine comfortably erect.

2. Tuck the chin by rotating the head forward on the top of the spine without bending the neck.

3. Bring the sternum up towards the chin, keeping the shoulders and back relaxed. If it touches, press the chest firmly against the chin.

4. Contract the throat.

Benefits of Jalandhara Bandha:

1. Regulates the flow of prana and blood to the head, preventing dizziness from pressure during breath retention.

2. Presses the ida and pingala nadis, locking the prana in the thorax, pressuring the prana to flow through the shushumna.

3. Clears the nasal passages of excess mucus.

Helpful Hints and Precautions:

The Chin Lock is performed during either internal or external retention of breath. With the Chin Lock you can hold your breath in without a feeling of pressure in the head. With the Chin Lock you can hold your breath out without a feeling of suction in your head.

Relax muscles not directly involved, such as face, jaw, tongue, shoulders, and back. As you practice this exercise the neck muscles will gradually become elongated and your chin will come down into the notch between the collarbones.

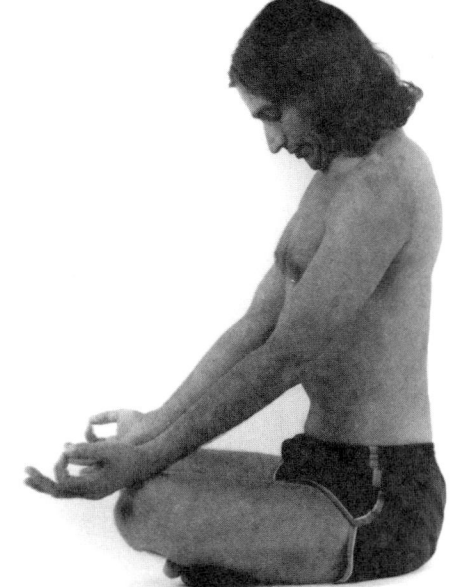

MULA BANDHA—ROOT LOCK

In the region below the navel, two-fingers-width above the midpoint of the perineum, lies the kanda or hara, where kundalini sleeps. Mula Bandha applies pressure and nurtures it with the energy that naturally goes with attention to this region during Mula Bandha, eventually awakening the sleeping energy.

Technique:

During pranayama use Mula Bandha in the following way:

1. Sit comfortably with the spine erect.

2. Place the left heel in the midpoint of the perineum, midway between the anus and the genitals. Apply pressure by placing your weight on your heel, to the extent this is comfortable.

3. Contract the perineum.

4. Pull the abdomen below the navel towards the spine. Keep the buttocks and upper abdomen relaxed.

5. Hold.

This lock can also be practiced in other postures.

Benefits of Mula Bandha:

1. This awakens the evolutionary energy called prana shakti.[1]

2. Prana is purified.

3. By pressing the ida and pingala, the prana is forced into the shushumna. That is the only open passageway left.

4. The practitioner experiences rejuvenation.

Helpful Hints and Precautions:

It may take some practice to isolate the muscles of the perineum. It may help to start by contracting the anus, then move the contraction forward. Keep the buttocks relaxed.

This posture may arouse strong energy in the muladhar chakra where it is experienced as sexual energy. The purpose of awakening the energy is not to indulge in sexual expression, but to raise it to higher consciousness through pranayama and meditation on the Third Eye (Ajna Chakra). Always keep the intensity of the energy at a level where the mind remains in control of the energy.

The same energy that habitually seeks outlet through sex, will, when raised and expressed through the heart, become the energy of pure love; when expressed through the Third Eye center, it will bestow the gift of non-attachment, fearlessness, objectivity, intuition, and wisdom. If you are unable to channel this energy towards the higher centers, discontinue the practice of Mula Bandha.

[1]See Book One.

ABDOMINAL EXTENSIONS

The purpose of this exercise is to release the muscular tensions held in the abdominal region. This exercise also helps facilitate the abdominal lifts, which are the opposite of the abdominal extensions.

Technique:

1. Lie comfortably in Shavasana (Corpse Pose): flat on your back, legs spread slightly apart, arms at your sides with palms up.

2. Bringing your concentration and awareness to the entire length and width of the abdomen (from below the ribs down to the pubis and over to the sides), inhale to between one-half and three-quarters of your full capacity as you expand the abdominal region fully.

3. Hold the breath in with this expansion for as long as comfortable.

4. Exhale and relax abdomen.

5. Repeat Steps 1-4 one to two more times.

6. Once again repeat Steps 1 and 2, this time pumping the abdomen in and out ten times while holding the breath in.

7. Exhale and relax abdomen.

8. Repeat Steps 1, 2, 6, 7 twice more.

9. Relax several moments, normalizing breath before going on to the next exercise.

Benefits of Abdominal Extensions:

1. Provides preparatory exercise for Uddiyana Bandha (Abdominal Lifts).

2. Stimulates digestion and elimination.

3. Removes tensions and blockages in the abdominal region.

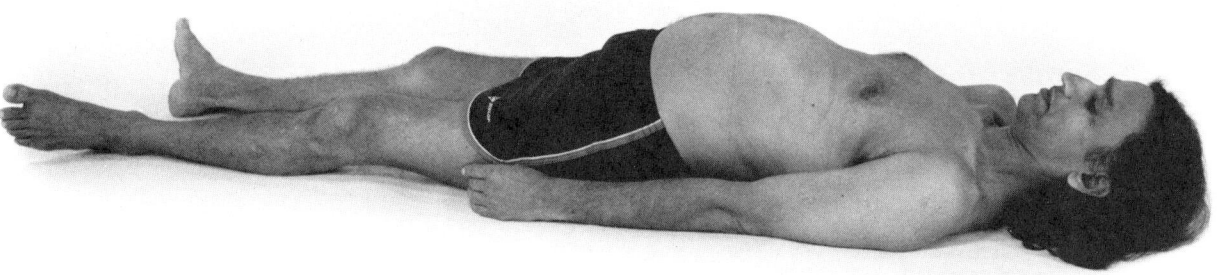

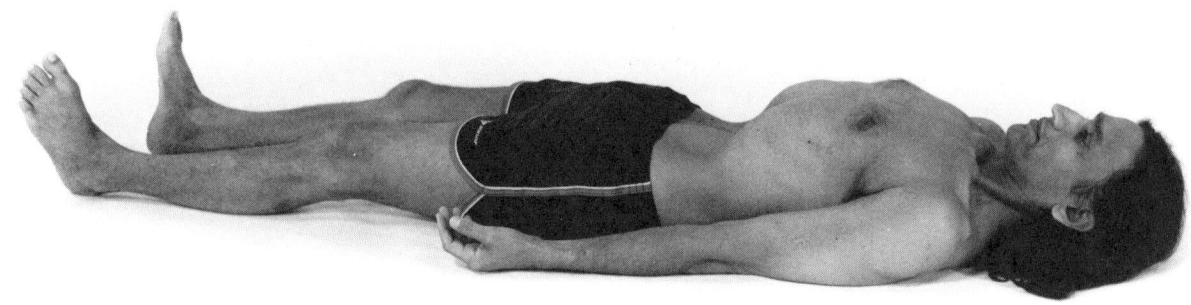

UDDIYANA BANDHA—ABDOMINAL LIFTS & AGNISARA DHAUTI—ABDOMINAL PUMPS

Technique:

1. Stand upright.

2. Spread legs about one foot apart.

3. Bend slightly forward from the waist and bend the knees slightly. Place the hands on the middle to lower thighs with the fingers either (a) spread wide on the middle of the thighs, or (b) turned towards the inner thighs.

4. Inhale deeply through the nostrils and then exhale quickly through the mouth so that all air is expelled from the lungs forcefully.

5. Hold the breath out without any inhalation.

6. Pull the whole abdominal region upward and back towards the spine. Pressing hands against the thighs helps contract the abdominal region and lift it up.

7. Maintain this Abdominal Lift, holding the breath for a moment before beginning Step 8. Continue to hold the breath.

8. Agnisara Dhauti (Abdominal Pumps): Allow the abdomen to return to normal position and then immediately pull it up again, and so on, pumping the abdomen twenty times.

9. Always rest between rounds, stabilizing the breath with Ujjayi (Sounding Breath) or Kapalabhati.

10. For present purposes, continue entire procedure for ten rounds with twenty abdominal pumps (Agnisara Dhauti) per round.

Benefits of Uddiyana Bandha and Agnisara Dhauti:

1. Exercises the diaphragm and abdominal organs.

2. Creates a cavity by the lift of the diaphragm that gives a gentle massage to the heart muscles, thereby toning the heart.

3. Tones abdominal organs.

4. Stimulates entire digestive tract through an increase in the power of digestion, thereby eliminating toxins from the tract.

5. Stimulates and decongests the liver, situated beneath the diaphragm.

6. Tones kidneys—increases diuretic action.

7. Stimulates adrenals.

8. Stimulates solar plexus area by stretching.

9. Stimulates lungs, bringing them greater elasticity.

Helpful Hints and Precautions:

Uddiyana Bandha is only to be performed during the interval between complete exhalation and fresh inhalation when breathing is suspended (Bahya Kumbhaka). Never perform Uddiyana Bandha during interval between complete inhalation and start of exhalation (Antara Kumbhaka). Do not practice Uddiyana Bandha while pregnant or menstruating.

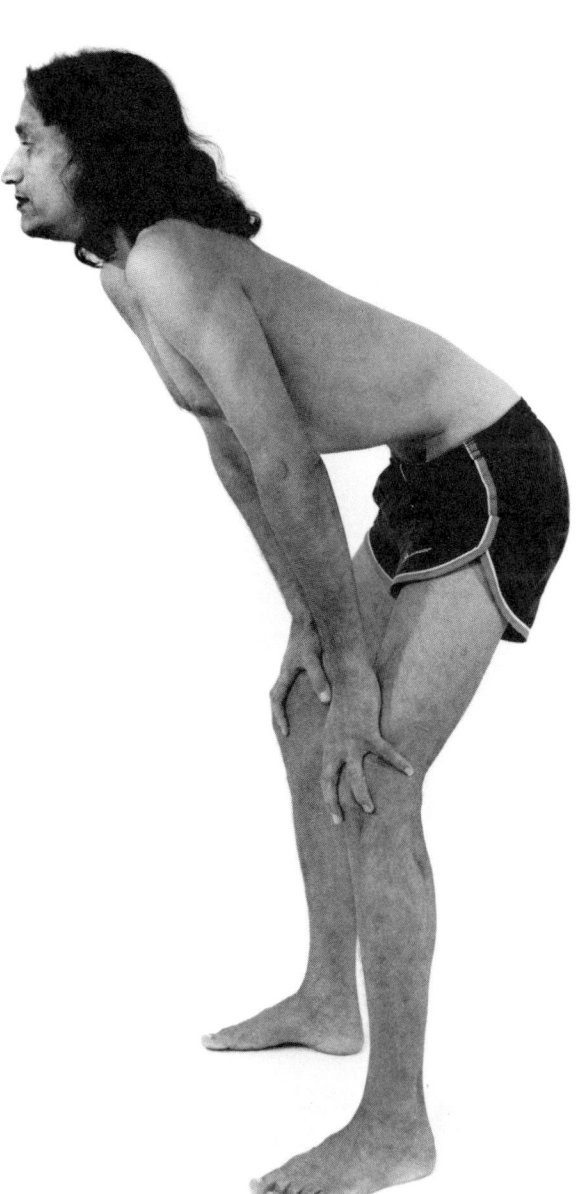

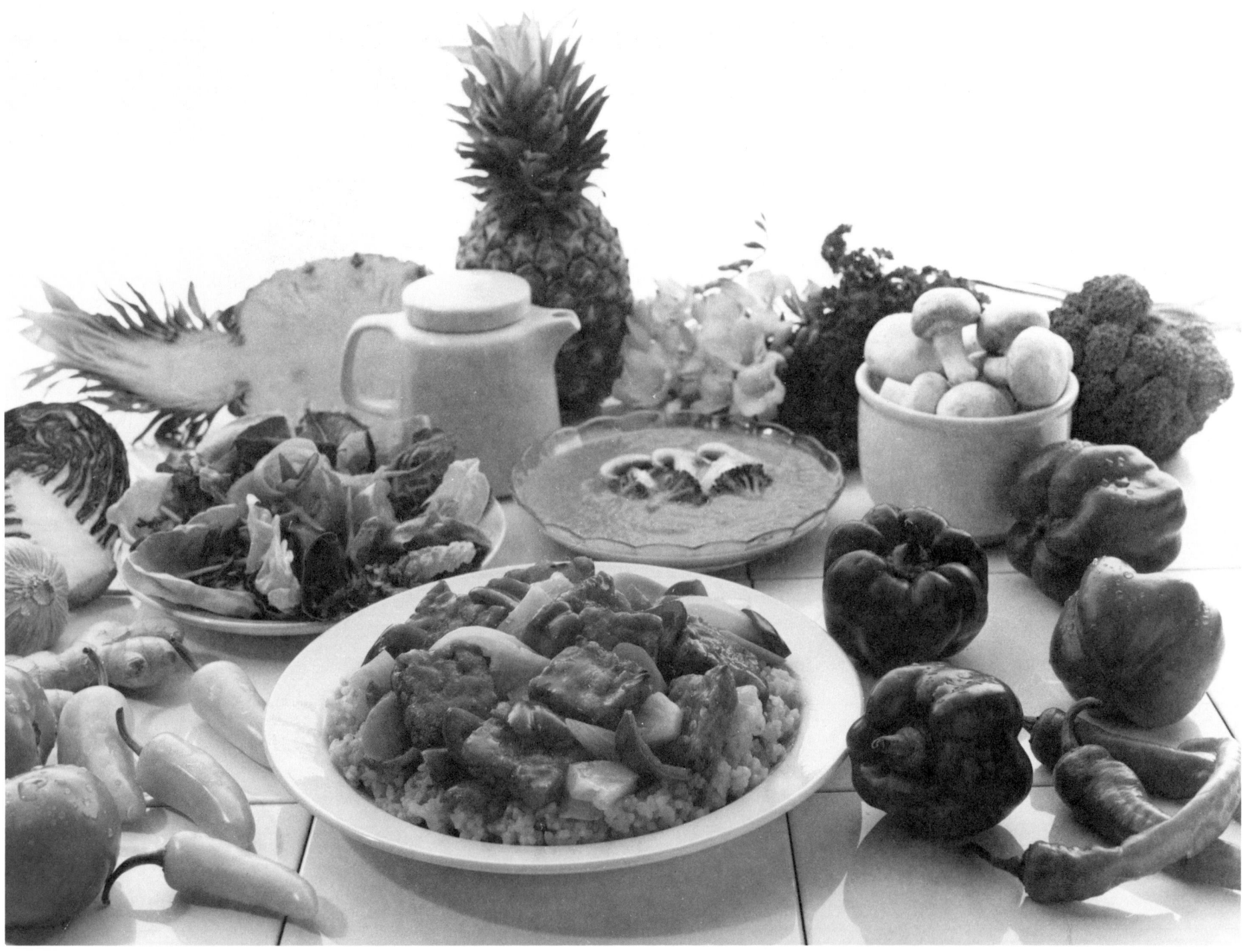

Diet

The Importance of Proper Diet

A nourishing balanced diet plays a crucial role in the successful practice of yoga postures, pranayama and meditation. The function of diet is to bring balance and energy into the body, which in turn reduces the restlessness of the mind, which is the basic purpose of yoga.

What you eat has a strong effect upon your mind. The great Masters of India and the East taught, thousands of years ago, that the body and mind are not two separate independent entities. Today a growing number of researchers are rediscovering that our emotions, moods, memory and our perceptions can be strongly influenced by what we eat.

A good diet is a natural and simple diet that supports and enhances yoga by eliminating foods that excessively stimulate the body and mind.

A Spiritual Diet

The most superb and healing diet for yoga that I have come across is what I call a **spiritual diet.** It is predominately whole grains, fresh cooked or raw vegetables, along with smaller portions of beans, legumes, fruits and nuts. Mainly in this diet you reduce the amount of salt, spices, and condiments, and reduce and possibly avoid sweeteners, refined flour products, oils and dairy products. What is detrimental, of course, is not so much what you eat from time to time, but what you eat regularly.

After I experimented with this diet, I was absolutely amazed by its profound impact. I derived great joy and deep satisfaction from my yoga. My mind became sharper and clearer than ever, body light, and my meditations became deeper. An inner sense of balance and harmony emerged that was more than just absence of disease or discomfort in the body. It is a superbly balanced diet. If an unhealthy person adopts it, he becomes healthy, and if the healthy person adopts it, it will speed up his spiritual growth.

SPIRITUAL DIET FOODS
Table One

Basic Foods	Occasional Foods	Foods to Avoid
Whole Grains	Whole Grain Flour	Refined Flour
Vegetables	Vegetable Juices	Processed Foods
Nuts & Seeds	Fruits	Canned Foods
Beans & Legumes	Dairy Products	Meat, Fish, Fowl
Herbal Teas	Vegetable Oils	Lard
Sea Vegetables	Salt and Spices	**Non-Foods to Avoid**
Miso, Tamari	Brewer's Yeast	Additives
Tofu, Tempeh	Barley Malt	Drugs, except
	Honey	essential prescriptions
	Maple Syrup	Alcohol
	Onions, Garlic	Caffein: coffee
	Tomatoes	chocolate, many colas,
	Potatoes	& black tea
		Nicotine
		Refined Sugar
		Preservatives

Any changes in diet should be made gradually to allow your body to adjust.

Moderation in Diet

Moderation in diet is essential in yoga. Even healthy food will, if overeaten, reduce your mental clarity and physical vitality. Bapuji defines moderate diet (mitahara) as "eating the precise amount of food required to keep the body alert and efficient."[1]

It is important to avoid eating more than a small amount of heavy, hard-to-digest foods. The imbalance caused by heavy undigested foods can cause mental and emotional stress.

Some form of vigorous physical activity must be made a part of our daily life to keep the appetite, digestion and elimination healthy. You will find that the quantity of food you are able to digest depends upon how much you exercise.

Conscious Eating

Conscious eating is learning to tune our mind into the wisdom of the body. Conscious eating means eating with full awareness of how, why, and what you are eating. It means slowing down and devoting your full attention during a meal to the experience of eating.

Always eat in a pleasant atmosphere. Begin your meal with a simple prayer of gratitude, or a moment of silence. This relaxes you and prepares your system to draw prana from the food you eat.

When you are eating, just eat. Try not to distract your attention and disturb your emotions with emotional news or scenes on TV or topics of conversation. Such activities distract you from the awareness that is necessary to chew food properly and taste it fully. When you do need to talk, make sure your conversation is gentle, pleasant and loving.

[1] Swami Kripalvanandji, *Pilgrimage of Love*, Book II, p. 221 (Kripalu Publications, 1982).

HIS HOLINESS SWAMI SHRI KRIPALVANANDJI

His Holiness Swami Shri Kripalvanandji (Bapuji) was one of the world's greatest masters of Kundalini yoga. For the last thirty years of his life, he devoted over 10 hours a day to the practice of Kundalini yoga meditation. As an example of his total dedication to this most arduous of spiritual practices, he missed only one day of meditation in this entire time—when he made his journey by airplane to the United States in 1977. For 22 of those years he practiced total silence, speaking only on rare public occasions.

Even though Bapuji was instrumental in establishing two major ashrams in India, his main focus was always his own personal sadhana (spiritual practices). Few truly great yogis have come to America; even fewer have chosen to come with such humility and self-effacement. After his arrival in 1977 Bapuji chose to live in seclusion at Kripalu Yoga Ashram in Sumneytown, Pennsylvania, founded and named in his honor by Yogi Amrit Desai. He returned to India in 1981, and entered Mahasamadhi (passed away) late that year.

A great poet, author, and classical musician, Bapuji spent most of his time when not in meditation in the activity of writing commentaries on the great yogic scriptures based upon his own personal experience of the higher practices of yoga.

Major works by Swami Kripalvanandji that have been translated into English are listed in the Bibliography. Major works in Gujarati include **Gitanjali,** a poetic rendition of the *Bhagavad-Gita;* **Asana and Mudra; Hatha Yoga Pradipika** commentary; and **Raga Jyoti,** a two volume work on classical Indian music. Books yet to be published are commentaries on *Patanjali's Yoga Sutras, Narad Bhakti Sutras,* and *Brahma Sutras,* all based upon his Kundalini yoga experiences.

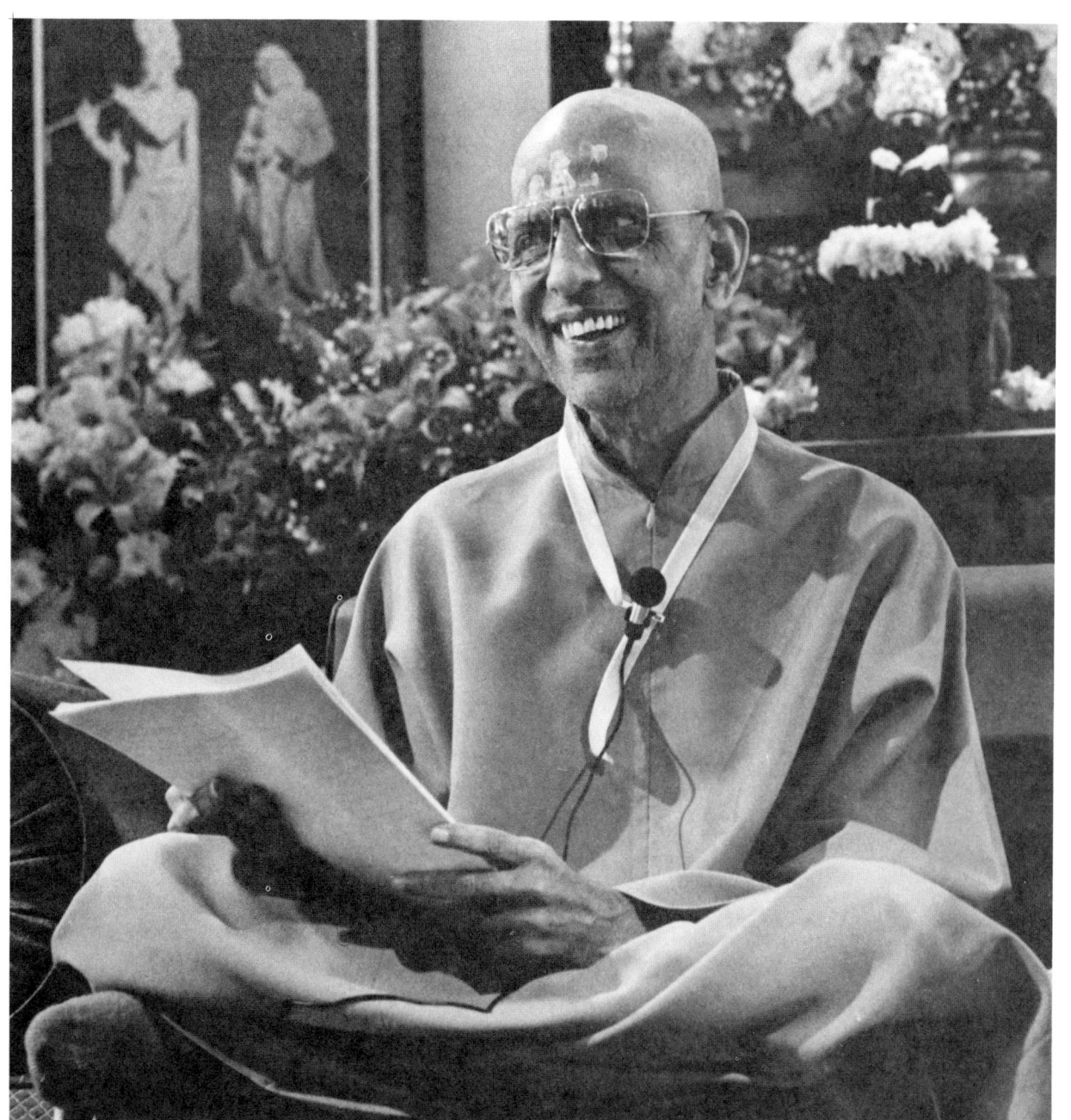

YOGI AMRIT DESAI

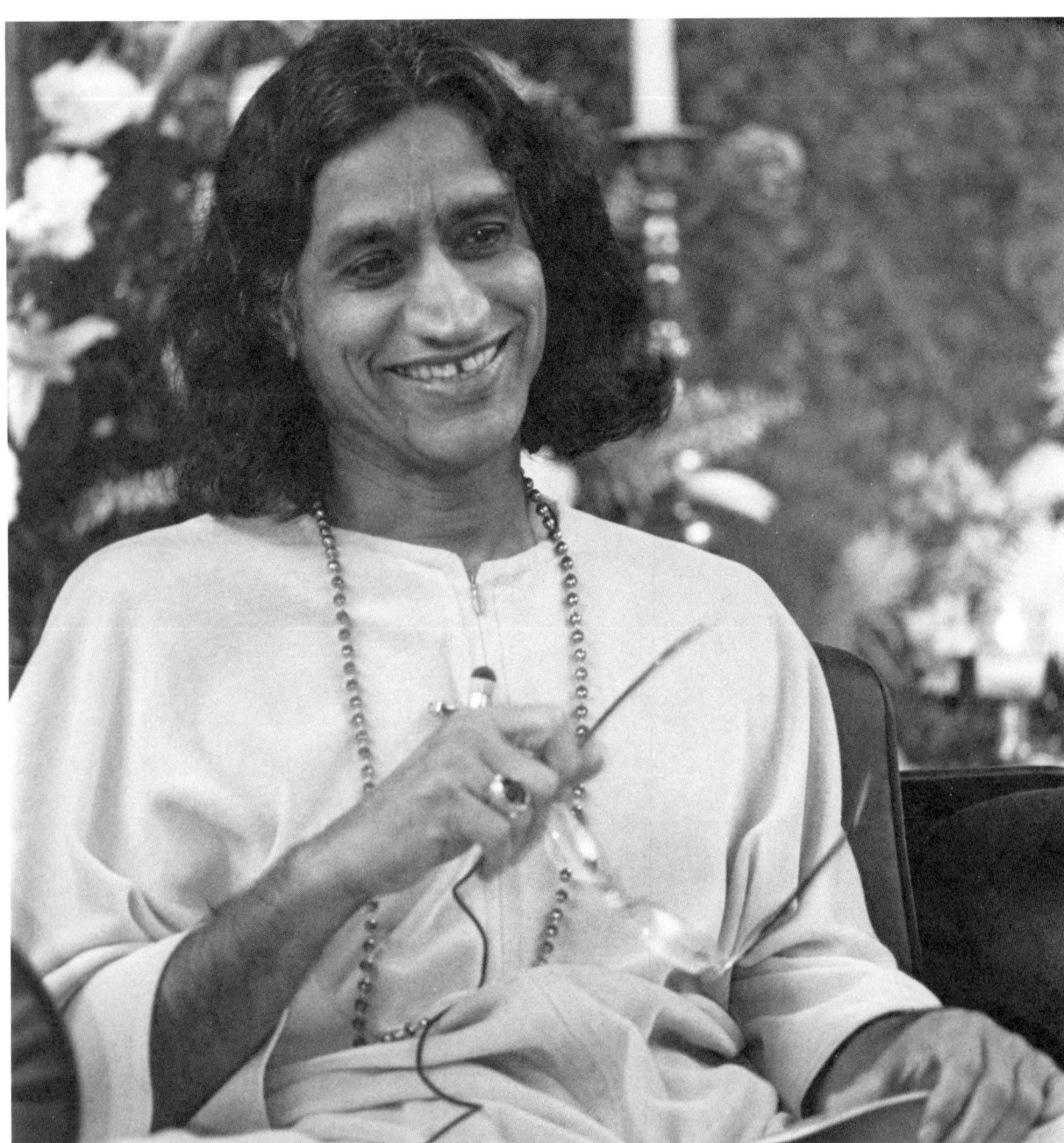

To be with Yogi Amrit Desai (often known as Gurudev) is, for many, an unforgettable experience. His is a strong, joyful, uplifting energy of love and wisdom. He feels like someone very familiar, very near and dear, even from the first encounter. His love, which he extends to each person he meets, has a child-like quality of openness and purity. His unconditional acceptance which is so obvious in both his life and his teachings, inspires love and trust.

Yogi Desai began yoga when he first met his guru, Swami Kripalvanandji in 1948 at the age of 16, but it was a profound spiritual experience in 1970 (described in this book) that transformed his life. Shortly afterwards, he received shaktipat initiation from his guru. Since then the energy awakened within him has had a powerful spiritual influence on the people who come close to him. That event marked the real beginning of his spiritual work, and this led to the development of Kripalu Yoga as well as Kripalu Yoga Ashram in 1970.

Yogi Desai says, "I was fortunate enough to be the disciple of one of the great Masters of India, Swami Kripalvanandji. He practiced Kundalini yoga meditation ten hours a day for the last thirty years of his life. He practiced total silence for twelve years; the last ten years he spoke publicly only twice a year. Through his rigorous sadhana of total dedication to God he reached to the highest stage of *Nirvikalpa Samadhi.* I was specially privileged to be one of his closest disciples, and to receive the most sacred gift of his spiritual heritage. He not only gave me *shaktipat diksha,* but he also empowered me to give shaktipat to sincere seekers to carry on this work in the West."

Yogi Desai is a universal teacher, and freely incorporates into his own teachings those of all masters and religions of the world. His words touch the hearts of people of all nationalities, religions, and walks of life. He is in demand as a speaker all over the world, and is the author of many books translated into several languages. Having been born in India, studied under a great Master, and taught for 25 years in the West, he is able to teach this secret wisdom of the East without losing the depth, quality, and purity of the ancient teachings. He teaches in practical terms that are easy to understand and to incorporate into the modern way of life.

His teachings come from his direct contact with his innermost being and knowing, and as a result are spontaneous, original, and universal. He speaks directly to the very core of our being. He says, "There is nothing I can teach you that you do not already know. All my teaching is but a reminder which your innermost knowing will confirm. In that sense, you already know what I have to say—yet these familiar ingredients combined in a new recipe that is a result of my direct realizations can become a source of new inspiration for you." His discourses have a way of speaking to the deepest questions of the heart, so that at the end each person feels "He was talking directly to me!" Thousands come to him and leave their problems at his feet, healed and refreshed by his presence and counsel.

Yogi Desai is an enlightened Master with penetrating insight and intuition. Whereas most of us may have a moment once in a while where we see to the core of reality, and sense the beauty, harmony, love, and unity behind the apparent diversity and disharmony, he lives in that perpetual awareness. Moreover, he has the ability to raise others to that state of consciousness and teach them how to integrate the experience into their lives so that they, too, can enter into similar levels of awareness. He does not personally claim any of this.

After his transforming experience in 1970, he went into seclusion to deepen his personal spiritual practices, but his loving nature and ability as a teacher attracted many sincere seekers who wanted to learn from him. Thus his sadhana became teaching and sharing with others rather than meditation in solitude. Since then he has dedicated his life to help others grow, and to see that happen is his greatest joy. Swami Kripalvanandji wrote about Yogi Desai: "If someone were to ask me, 'Among your householder disciples[1], whom do you consider most evolved?' I would definitely nominate Amrit first! Amrit is extremely loving; he is fond of sadhana and loves the saints and the scriptures; and he has invoked love for his guru in the hearts of thousands of disciples. His life is like that of a saint."

Yogi Desai has created and directed several ashrams and health centers. The first Ashram was born in 1970. The number of ashram residents grew steadily and to accommodate the growing number of seekers, a larger second Yoga Retreat was acquired in 1975 near Summit Station, Pennsylvania. There, in 1979, Yogi Desai created the Holistic Health Center which has grown into one of the largest and finest of its kind in the country. In 1983, to accommodate growing demands, the present Kripalu Center for Yoga and Health was established in Stockbridge, Massachusetts, which can accommodate 230 staff and nearly 400 guests. It offers a wide range of programs in yoga, holistic health, and personal growth, serving thousands of guests each year. It has 45 branches in North America, Europe, and India.

Yogi Desai has been honored repeatedly by the spiritual leaders of India and by the American academic community for his mastery of yoga, for his remarkable accomplishments as a spiritual teacher, and for his service to humanity. His Holiness Jagadguru Shankaracharya, one of the foremost spiritual authorities in India, conferred on him an honorary Doctor of Yogic Science degree (1974) in appreciation of his outstanding contributions to humanity and his knowledge of yoga. He was also awarded the title Acharya Pravaraha (Supreme Spiritual Teacher) (1975) by Swami Vedavyasanandji, Chancellor of Rishikul Sanskrit University in Haridwar, India. The title Yogacharya (Spiritual Preceptor) (1980) was conferred by His Holiness Swami Shri Kripalvanandji in honor of his mastery in teaching the spiritual principles and the practices of yoga. He was also given the title Maharishi (Great Sage) (1982) by his Holiness Swami Shri Gangeshwaranandji Udasin, 102 year-old spiritual preceptor, who is highly revered throughout India. In spite of these and other titles, he typically prefers to be called simply Gurudev or Yogi Desai.

Yogi Desai once said:

"I have not come to teach you,
but to love you;
love itself will teach you."

His life and works affirm these words.

---

[1]Yogi Desai has a wife and three children.

KRIPALU CENTER

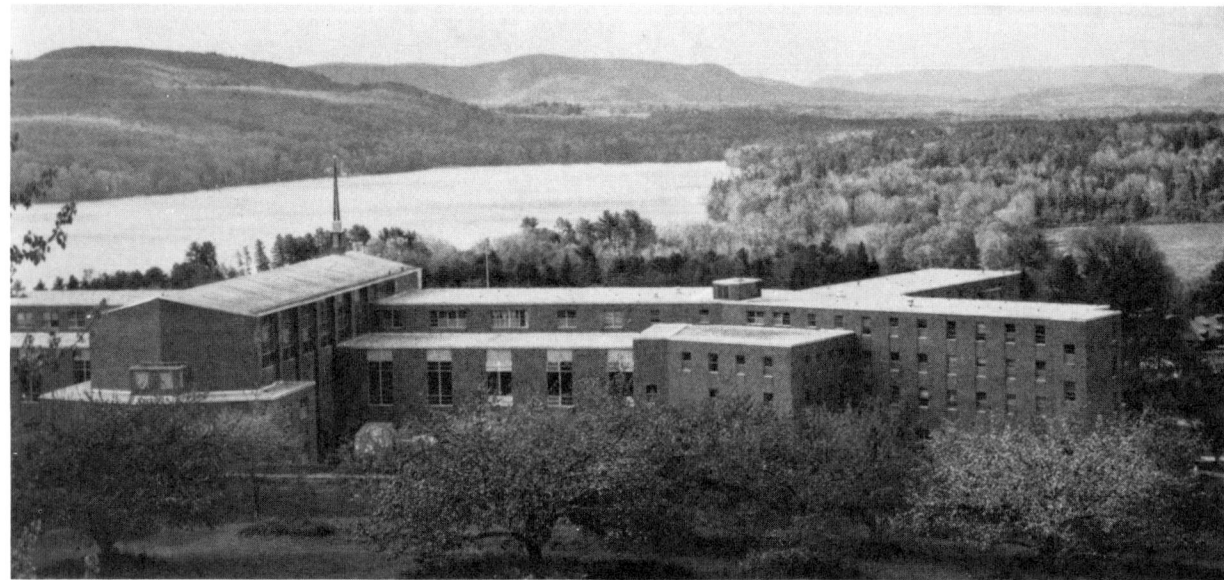

The fundamental approach of Kripalu Center is loving service to others. As Yogi Desai describes it:

Our purpose is to help people, but it goes deeper than that. "Service to humanity" remains a barren, idealistic action if it does not also serve your inborn need to grow. If you establish the attitude that everything in the business of your daily life has the potential to teach you about life, then every experience whether pleasure or pain, success or failure, comes with a message that relates to your inner growth.

That orientation to spiritual growth has been the byword for Kripalu's growth. The present organization has evolved in its 20-year history into an independent non-profit federally tax-exempt corporation which is the parent of activities in Massachusetts, and also of a small, flourishing residential community in the original location in Sumneytown, Pennsylvania. The physical facilities of Kripalu Center are located on beautiful Lake Mahkeenac in the Berkshire mountains, in western Massachusetts. The main building, which has over four acres of floor space and 400 rooms, houses the resident staff of over 200, as well as program guests.

Activities at Kripalu Center

Yogi Desai teaches resident staff that true learning is experiential, and that we can only truly teach that which we live in everyday life. As a result, Kripalu provides both staff and guests a supportive environment which models the health and transformation principles it teaches. Guests may, if they choose, participate fully in the holistic lifestyle that has been developed over the years by the resident staff.

Group programs at Kripalu Center—weekend, week-long, or month-long—are educational and transformational in nature. These programs provide both experiential learning and practical methods for a way of life which integrates body, mind, and spirit into one harmonious whole.

Guests, no matter what their background or work, can apply these powerful growth experiences to enrich their daily lives. According to their primary emphasis, our programs focus on: Health and Fitness, Self-Discovery, Yoga, Spiritual Attunement, Bodywork Training, and Month-Long Professional Training.

Each program is open to people with all levels of experience, unless it is an advanced course in a series. As a guest, you may want to select a program that addresses a particular interest. Accordingly, we have grouped our programs into several categories depending upon their primary focus.

In programs with a focus on:	you experience how to:
Health and Fitness	promote your body's power to heal itself; move beyond unhealthy habits to a lifestyle which generates well-being.
Self-Discovery	observe and transform the patterns of thinking and feeling that condition your relationship to yourself and others.
Yoga	use the body as a vehicle to raise and center your energy; discard self-imposed limitations in body and mind and help others do the same.
Spiritual Attunement	invoke the wisdom that comes to you with inner stillness; draw upon this innate knowing for consistent inspiration.
Bodywork Training	activate your healing energy to enhance your own health, and help others as well, with a variety of hands-on techniques.

The daily schedule for guests includes three vegetarian meals, classes in yoga, relaxation, and Kripalu® DansKinetics, plus workshops tailored for the particular program. Private, double-occupancy, and dormitory accommodations are available; a program for children is open during the summer season. Guests and residents alike enjoy year-round sauna and whirlpool facilities, as well as hikes, swimming, or skiing on the spacious and beautiful 300+ acres surrounding the Center.

As a guest, your experience at Kripalu Center is a montage of discoveries: ideas and skills, facilities and events, feelings and friendships.

At Kripalu Center, guests experience what loving their whole self means. And that experience doesn't end when they leave. While they are here, they learn practical ways to keep that loving feeling going and growing, wherever they are. Freeing your self, freeing your love to grow: that's self-transformation. That's what the Kripalu experience is all about.

Yoga Teacher Training

This comprehensive training program offers detailed instruction in the theory, practice, application, and benefits of the Kripalu approach to the fundamental yoga postures (asanas) and breathing techniques (pranayama) that form the basis for living and teaching a yogic lifestyle.

Our training methods have evolved over years of experience and allow you to develop your own natural teaching style. Practice teaching, personal growth experiences, and guided self-reflection exercises are all included in your training to help increase your self-understanding and to enable you to communicate to those you teach with insight, confidence, and proficiency.

The month of training includes studies in the philosophy and psychology of yoga and in the teachings of Yogi Desai. Of special importance are the times spent in sessions with Yogi Desai when he is in residence.

You receive step-by-step lesson plans and learn how to tailor your yoga classes to special audiences and settings. When you leave, you will know who to contact and how to promote your services as a yoga teacher in your community.

To receive teaching certification, one year's practice of hatha yoga is required. Those not meeting this prerequisite may enroll for personal interest; their certification will be deferred until they complete one year's practice.

All Kripalu programs shift consciousness back to the body and highlight the need to balance energies and improve one's health as a prerequisite for achieving the peace and personal transformation or spiritual growth that is necessary for effective service to others. The Kripalu approach, truly holistic in nature, helps people tap their inner resources and lead fuller, happier lives. Living life as an art is the highest experience. As Yogi Desai puts it:

When you consciously create your life, then you are an artist in the true sense of the word. Yes, I gave up my career as an artist, but only to practice the highest of arts: the art of living. To share this art with others is my greatest joy.

For more information on our calendar of programs, write or call: **Kripalu Center, P.O. Box 793, Lenox, MA 01240, (413) 637-3280.**

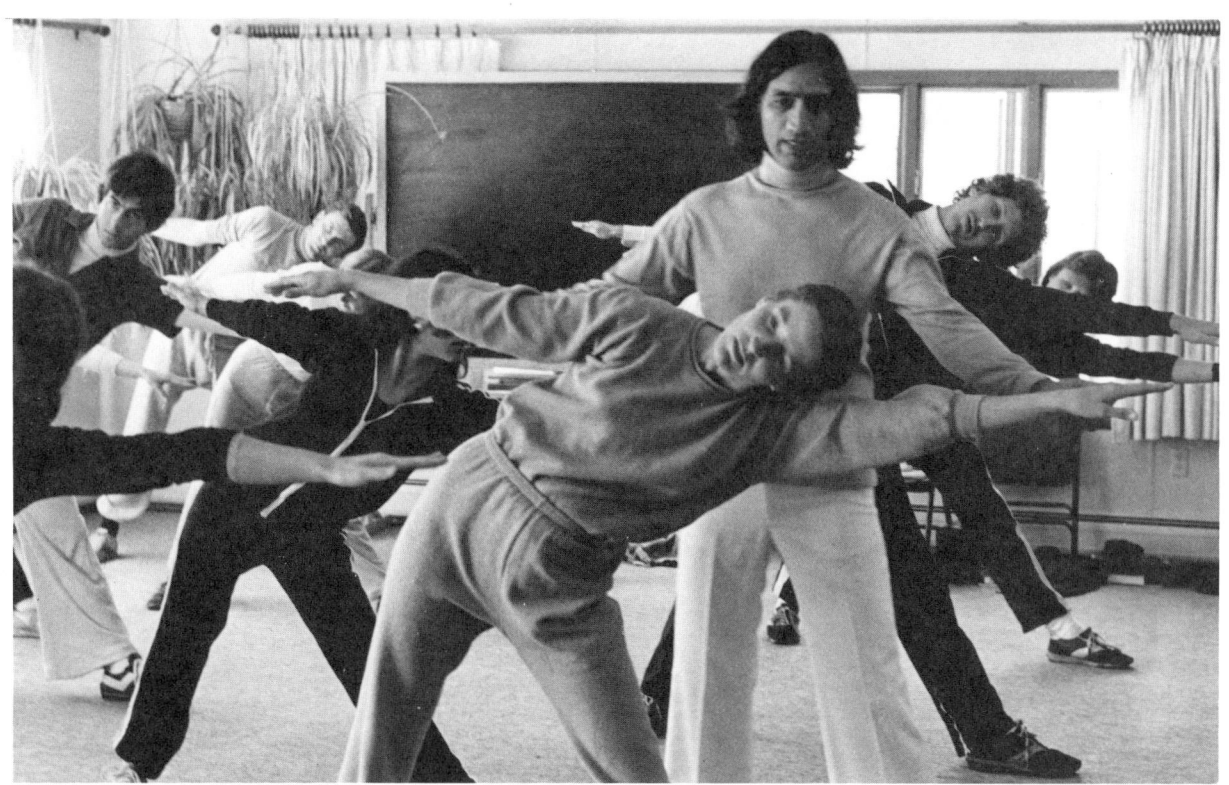

TABLE OF CONTENTS OF BOOK I

BIBLIOGRAPHY

KRIPALU PUBLICATIONS

Desai, Yogi Amrit

Kripalu Yoga: Meditation-in-Motion (1981); Revised & Enlarged Edition, (1985).

Happiness Is Now: Reflective Writings of Yogi Amrit Desai (1982).

The Wisdom of the Body (1984).

Working Miracles of Love (1985). *Collection of shorter works.*

Love is an Awakening (1985).

Kripalvanandji, Yogacharya Swami

Premyatra: A Pilgrimage of Love, Book I (1981).

Premyatra: A Pilgrimage of Love, Book II (1982).

Premyatra: A Pilgrimage of Love, Book III (1984).

Warren, Sukanya; Frances Mellen; and Peter Mellen

Gurudev: The Life of Yogi Amrit Desai (1982).

BOOKS DISTRIBUTED BY KRIPALU CENTER

Kripalvanandji, Yogacharya Swami

Science of Meditation (1977).

Muni, Rajarshi

Light from Guru to Disciple (1974).

BOOKS AVAILABLE FROM KRIPALU CENTER

Pradhan, V. G. (Translator); Lambert, H. M. (Editor)

Jnaneshwari (Bhavarthadipika); a commentary by Jnanadeva on the **Bhagavadgita** (London: George Allen Unwin, Ltd., 1967), Volumes I and II.

Taimni, I. K.

The Science of Yoga; a commentary on the **Yoga Sutras** of Patanjali (Wheaton, Illinois: Theosophical Publishing House, 1975).

OTHER RELEVANT READING

Bernard, Theos

Hatha Yoga: The Report of a Personal Experience (New York: Samuel Weiser, 1947). *Out-of-print.*

Hindu Philosophy (Bombay, India: Jaico Publishing House, 125 Mahatma Gandhi Road, 1958, 1964), pp. 84-103. *Out-of-print.*

Gallwey, W. Timothy

The Inner Game of Tennis (New York: Bantam Books, 1982).

Gallwey, Timothy, and Bob Kriegel

Inner Skiing (New York: Bantam Books, 1981).

Kripalvanandji, Yogacharya Swami

Asana & Mudra (In Gujarati; 1967).

The Sadhak's Companion (1977).

Leonard, George

The Silent Pulse (New York: Bantam Books, 1981).

Maslow, Abraham H.

Toward a Psychology of Being (2nd ed. New York: Van Nostrand Reinhold Company, 1968).

McCluggage, Denise

The Centered Skier (Revised ed. New York: Bantam Books, 1983).

Murphy, Michael, and Rhea A. White

The Psychic Side of Sports (Reading, Massachusetts: Addison-Wesley Publishing Company, 1978).

Singh, Pancham (Translator)

Hatha Yoga Pradipika (New Delhi, India: Munishiram Manoharlal Publishers, 1980).

Tirtha, Swami Vishnu

Devatma Shakti (Kundalini) Divine Power (Rishikesh, India: Swami Shivom Tirth, 1974).

Index